Eat Complete

Also by Drew Ramsey, MD

Fifty Shades of Kale
The Happiness Diet

Eat Complete

The 21 Nutrients That **Fuel Brainpower, Boost Weight Loss**, and **Transform** Your **Health**

Drew Ramsey, MD

HARPER WAVE

An Imprint of HarperCollinsPublishers

EAT COMPLETE. Copyright © 2016 by Drew Ramsey. All rights reserved. Printed in the United States of America. No part of this book may be used or reproduced in any manner whatsoever without written permission except in the case of brief quotations embodied in critical articles and reviews. For information, address HarperCollins Publishers, 195 Broadway, New York, NY 10007.

HarperCollins books may be purchased for educational, business, or sales promotional use. For information, please e-mail the Special Markets Department at SPsales@harper collins.com.

FIRST EDITION

All photographs by Ellen Silverman

Linen photograph by Hellen Sergeyera/Shutterstock, Inc.

Designed by Leah Carlson-Stanisic

Library of Congress Cataloging-in-Publication Data has been applied for.

ISBN: 978-0-06-241343-7

19 20 21 22   LSCC   10 9 8 7 6 5 4

To Lucy, Greta, and Forrest.
No meal is complete without you.

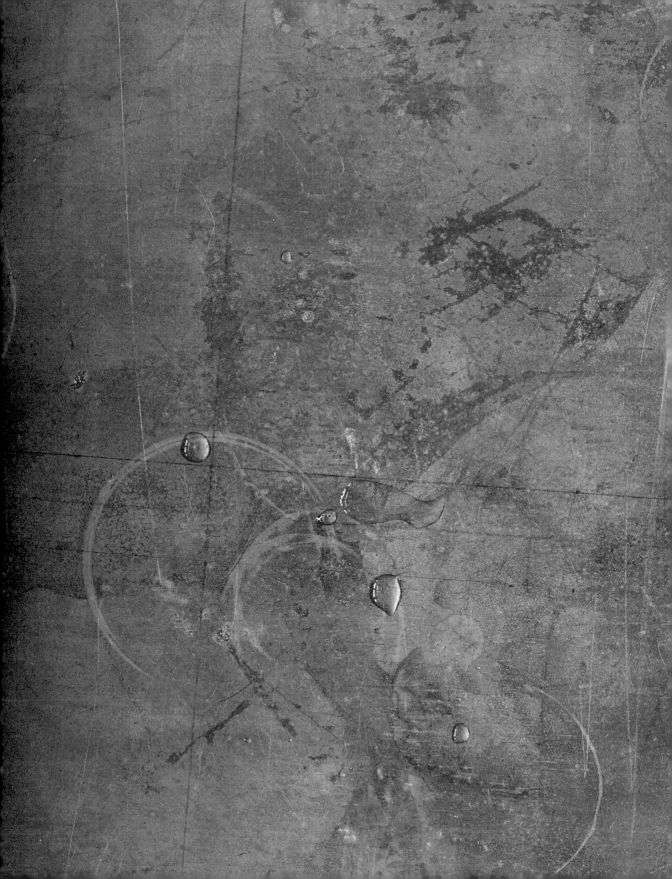

Contents

Eat Complete

A Doctor Learns to PRESCRIBE FOOD

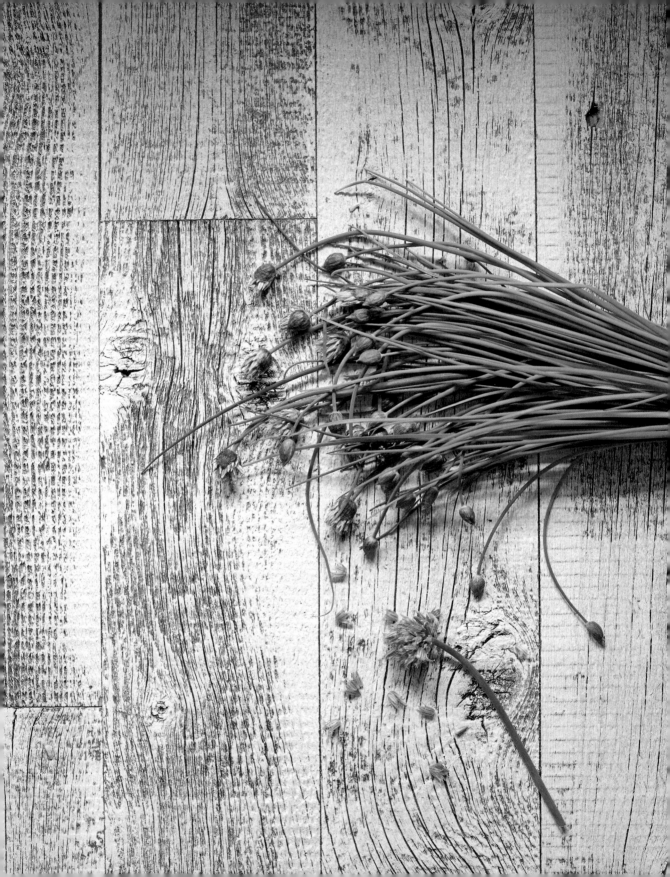

Our health is being challenged like never before in history. You've seen the headlines: modern food and lifestyle have made us sick, a nation over-fed and yet undernourished. Add to this the new stressors of ceaseless media, more work, and less sleep. The need for proper nourishment and self-care is pressing and unprecedented.

Thankfully, the foundation of good health is delicious. For the first time in centuries, doctors are prescribing food. As our focus on health, nutrition, and wellness has grown, so too has the role of food in medicine. My work as a psychiatrist is all about brain health, which means helping people care for and protect their biggest asset: the brain. And it turns out that brain health is directly influenced by the food we eat.

Nutritional psychiatry is the new forefront of the psychiatric field, a movement focused on the mental health impact of food. As the movement has grown, so too has my desire to bring the important lessons about the impact of food on the brain to a wider audience. The advice in these pages is a prescription for

your brain health and wellness, intended to help you cut through the controversies and eat with confidence. And the best prescription is to feed your brain properly, as an undernourished brain has profound implications for all aspects of life.

I learned about food growing up on my family's farm in southern Indiana, and I learned about brain health at Columbia University College of Physicians and Surgeons, the top department of psychiatry in the United States, where I trained and have taught for the last twelve years. I now teach brain nutrition to graduate students and psychiatry residents, and I'm also in active clinical practice doing my best to apply my training to the art of medicine. While I primarily treat patients with mood and anxiety disorders, this book is for the general public. **Everyone with a brain should know how to feed it.**

A few years back, I changed how I practice medicine. A new class of medications was causing a series of side effects for the patients in our clinic. While these medications were often necessary, patients began to gain weight at an alarming rate, and frequently developed diabetes and high blood pressure. As a physician bound to the maxim "Do no harm," I am obligated to help mediate these side effects. Healthy eating and exercise were major interests in my personal life, and I'd been a vegetarian for about a decade, but I hadn't been talking to my patients about food and lifestyle choices.

It started to gnaw at me. Not only were the medications I was prescribing adding to my patients' health problems, but I realized I was totally untrained to counsel them about nutrition. Doctors don't learn about nutrition in medical school, even though poor food choices are at the root of the majority of health concerns in our country. I remember sitting with a woman who was free of the symptoms of her mental illness for the first time in years, realizing that she had also gained thirty pounds. I knew then that food needed to be a fundamental part of our assessment and prescription as doctors.

Food became a focus of my work. Increasingly curious about what my patients ate, I was also determined to find out what I should advise them to eat based on scientific evidence. I started talking to patients about their food, and reading about the recent advances in the science of nutrition. I learned that my patients were just as confused as I was. I felt foolish as I realized that the standard advice I was offering—"Don't eat cholesterol or fat"—was both scientifically wrong and woefully inadequate. I also learned that my vegetarian diet wasn't likely the healthiest. It was time to figure out what constituted a healthy meal.

As my understanding of healthy foods captivated my work as a physician, it also took a prominent role in my personal life thanks to a new motivation: my wife was pregnant with our daughter. Every molecule in our daughter's developing brain would come from the food choices we made over the next few years. I needed to establish a core set of foods that would best nourish our new family.

As a physician interested in brain health, I've been struck by how little we consider the impact of food. We think of our bodies, but we put minimal thought and focus into how food choices relate to our brains, or how the state of our brains can affect so many important aspects of our overall health and mood. Our brains are both our greatest asset and the home of the hungriest cells in our body. It's crucial to feed these cells well—and that's important across the board, whether or not you are a patient on my couch. Not matter your personal background, genetics, or situation, the core of your personal wellness is your food.

As the science continues to advance, it's become easier to see the impact food has on our brain health. Our brains consume 20 percent of everything we eat; this nourishment provides the energy and nutrients to create and sustain the quadrillions of connections that construct the brain, and the electricity that courses between those connections. Your brain is the organ of connection, and you depend on these connections for all aspects of your life: Your work. Your relationships. Your memories. Your intentions. Your dreams. You have in your possession the most complex structure in the known universe, a human brain—but most of us, myself included, were never taught how to optimally fuel it.

In my practice, I was prescribing medications and doing talk therapy, but it seemed clear that food presented a unique opportunity to further help my patients. It would certainly be my most delicious prescription. Better food choices would

ensure that my patients' brains were optimally nourished with "building block" nutrients such as omega-3 fats, vitamin B_{12}, and zinc. It would also make their brains more resilient by enhancing brain growth—the latest brain science tells us that human brains continue to grow through adulthood, creating new brain cells and also new connections. On top of that, eating better food would decrease my patients' risk of obesity, diabetes, and heart disease, all diseases that wreak havoc on mental health.

Armed with this knowledge, I made "food as medicine" the primary focus of my clinical work. My colleagues and I started to serve the patients in our clinic more plants and other nutrient-rich foods for lunch. Many started to lose weight and reported an improvement in their mood and self-confidence. This became a key tool in their treatment. And in addition to better nourishment, they also engaged in the mindful art of self-care.

My goal today is to help people achieve proper nourishment with every bite—and it's become clear from the results that food can be an excellent medicine. Recently, a patient with panic attacks was largely cured by eating more seafood and having eggs for breakfast. A woman in her thirties noticed a significant reduction in her severe anxiety and mood swings after introducing more seafood and lentils into her food plan. A teenager who was irritable and argumentative with his parents became more reasonable with them after starting his day with a fruit, yogurt, and nut smoothie.

After I saw significant positive results like these, my first line of defense for patients became their nutrition. I now complete a nutrition assessment during my initial evaluations of patients, along with a brain food prescription. Food remains part of my ongoing clinical conversation, and I consider nutrition to be a key aspect of my clinical work overall. Helping people fully fuel their brains and eat foods that promote

stable moods, clear thinking, and a more resilient brain just makes sense.

And it makes sense for everyone, not just my patients. The building blocks of your brain—all the vitamins, minerals, fats, sugars, and proteins—start at the end of your fork. Your eating pattern dictates the health and function of your brain, as well as the rate of your brain's growth. That is what inspired me to write this cookbook. Most people don't think about nutrition, and certainly not about how nutrition affects the brain. But it's time to end eating confusion—and, while we're at it, boost the power of our brains.

CHAPTER ONE

What Does It Mean to
EAT COMPLETE?

The key to a healthy brain and body—and therefore optimal health—is to "eat complete." Eating complete means that you get all of the nutrients your brain and body need from the food you eat. But for many people, it's challenging to focus on nutrition in a way that is feasible, convenient, and delicious. Instead, it's easy to make poor choices, fall into bad food habits, and often leave out the very foods we need most in our diets.

As I began addressing food and nutrition with the patients in my clinical practice, I found myself running into three common barriers. The first is that it is complicated for people to eat in a way that optimizes nutrients. How do you know what to do, and who can you trust about food? Another barrier comes from concerns about time and money. Many people feel they lack the skills and time to cook every night, and healthy food can be expensive. Finally, in order to work around these other two barriers, people often put blind trust in a bad insurance policy: the daily multivitamin. The data on supplementation are mixed at best—but either way, there is no insurance policy for eating poorly.

The more I ran into these barriers, the more I focused on helping my patients overcome them. Over the years of assessing people's food habits, a pattern of missing nutrients became apparent to me. In conjunction, there has been a surge in the scientific evidence about brain health and nutrition (more on this below). Recent studies have looked at dietary patterns and the risk of brain-based illnesses such as depression and dementia, and the results are showing strong correlations between those illnesses and what we eat. Coupled with the modern discovery that the human brain is growing even in adulthood, the conclusions are startling. The very nutrients many people are missing are those most important to human brain health. And without these nutrients, your brain and body will not operate as they should.

Take, for example, the brain chemical serotonin, which regulates critical physiology such as mood, weight, and sex drive. For your brain to produce this chemical, you must eat foods that contain the amino acid tryptophan (such as pumpkin seeds, cod, and beef) as well as foods high in iron, folate, and vitamin B_{12} (such as lentils, mussels, and kale). While many foods contain these nutrients, only a few contain enough to help you meet the required daily dose.

The more I learned about the nutritional needs of the body, and especially those of the brain, the more I began to wonder—was it even possible to obtain all of the nutrients you need from food? For example, human health depends on getting at least 400 milligrams of magnesium every day. Where do you find it? I didn't know. Neither did my colleagues. And my patients certainly didn't know either.

So back to the main question: Can you actually get the most important nutrients for your health, such as magnesium, just by eating food? The answer is yes—it just takes a little knowledge, a core set of foods, and

100 recipes to get you started. And that's the goal of *Eat Complete*.

The 21 Nutrients of Transformation

The 21 nutrients (vitamins, minerals, fats, protein, plant-based phytonutrients, and health-promoting bacteria) that form the core of this book come from the rapidly evolving science of how food changes the brain. I've selected them based on this science, and on the reality that Americans are missing a number of key nutrients in their diets. The simple and scary truth is that the majority of Americans eat a diet that is lacking the most important nutrients for health. Recent data from the United States Department of Agriculture (USDA) found that most people are not meeting the Recommended Daily Allowance for many key nutrients. For example, 68 percent of people are not getting enough magnesium, 75 percent are not getting enough folate, and a whopping 86 percent are not getting enough vitamin E.

In the following pages, I'll explain why these 21 nutrients are the core of living a healthy life. I'll review each of the nutrients in detail, and I'll also show you how to incorporate high concentrations of these nutrients into your diet with whole, natural foods and simple, delicious recipes. These tasty meals will fuel your brain, keep your body lean, and transform your health.

Focusing on the foods that maximize these 21 nutrients ensures your meals are rich in the compounds most important for your success. The foods you eat help build and fuel your brain, allowing it to make new connections and even signal the birth of new brain cells. When you feed your brain the most important nutrients with the minimal number of calories, your brain will function better and you will be your optimal weight. A healthy brain offers protection from low moods and anxiety, as well as better resilience during times of stress. And having a sharper, happier, and more resilient brain is ultimately what it takes to transform your overall health.

Additionally, when you eat the whole healthy foods that contain these nutrients, you will avoid a number of ingredients in modern food that are horrible for your health, such as trans fats, artificial food dyes, preservatives, pesticides, and persistent organic pollutants—all of which are tied to brain health problems and weight gain. One reason we are so undernourished and yet overfed is that we're using the wrong foods as fuel.

There is a lot of hyperbole in the health and wellness scene, but it is not my intention to add to that. If I seem optimistic about your health, it is for a good reason.

Over the last fifteen years as a physician, I've seen a lot of people radically change their lives. When intention is aligned with a commitment to self-care, the human spirit is an unstoppable force. Transformations happen when a brain is at full power and a person is at a healthy weight. These two factors—brain power and a healthy weight— are what these recipes are designed to deliver. Eat your way to a better brain and body, and transform your health by eating complete.

Building a Tool Kit: Arming Yourself with Knowledge

Over the last few decades, we have dissected our food and eating habits as never before in history. Such scrutiny has led to a number of trends. In my work, I come across eaters of every stripe: The Paleo tribe. Vegans. Pescatarians. Fasters. Juicers. Jenny Craigers. Weight Watchers. It's clear that having a set of rules for eating helps people.

Eating complete doesn't have to replace those rules. Part of the challenge of good nutritional advice is the art of guiding people to their goal, helping them find a place where they are content and satisfied.

That's a unique place for each of us, as we each have our own palate and our own set of values that guide our eating. To cater to as many eaters as possible, almost all of the recipes in this book have optional (and easy) modifications for everyone from vegans to Paleos. Almost all the recipes are naturally gluten-free, and the few that aren't will surprise you by showing you how fermenting flour as sourdough greatly reduces the gluten.

My role here first and foremost is to be a resource for you. With so much debate about nutrition, people often have no idea that when it comes to your brain, eating a plant-based diet is great, but eating only plants equals malnutrition. After all, this is why strict vegans are obligated to take supplements. While there are plenty of plant-worshipping vegan dishes in this book, I have also consciously selected seafood and meat dishes that would serve as the best invitation to the vegan and vegetarian readers looking to expand their palates.

By asking you to make the idea of "fueling your brain" your primary goal as an eater, I'm asking you to take a step back and look at your food through a different lens. This means reconsidering how you think about food and nutrition. For example, fat, a perpetual enemy of "healthy" eating for decades, is actually at the top of the list of nutrients for a healthy brain and body. It's

also worth calling attention to the phrase "plant-based diet." This means most of your plate is made up of vegetables, nuts, beans, fruits, and whole grains. But all diets on the planet are currently plant based, as photosynthesis in plants and in algae is at the base of the food supply. Without plants and photosynthesis, we'd have no food. But eating *only* plants is often portrayed as a healthy diet, when it actually leads to nutrient deficiencies of vitamin B$_{12}$, long-chained omega-3 fats, and often iron and zinc. Furthermore, not all plants are created equal. After all, three plants—sugarcane, corn, and soybeans—are at the heart of our country's nutrition problems thanks to their role as the primary ingredients in most processed foods.

It's also imperative to understand that the real toxins in food are more than just sugar, refined carbs, or gluten. Not only are we often demonizing the wrong foods, but we're ignoring the fact that modern food contains some strange new molecules that humans have never eaten. Research on the negative health effects of food dyes, brominated compounds, and fake fats is compelling enough that I've banned them from my family's kitchen. The FDA plans to eliminate trans fats from the food supply by 2018, but you can eliminate them now by avoiding highly processed, packaged foods. Such a move would also largely help eliminate your exposure to toxins such as plasticizers, persistent organic pollutants, and synthetic estrogens, all of which throw our metabolism and health out of balance by acting as endocrine disrupters.

My hope is that this book will encourage you to confidently explore a new set of foundational foods that can get you started on this journey towards health and happiness. The following pages will arm you with a new set of moves in the kitchen, along with some facts and figures that will change the way you fill your refrigerator. For example, the top source of vitamin B_{12} is clams. Smaller fruits have more nutrients. Grass-fed beef has a healthier nutritional profile than chicken. The right choice in chocolate could enhance your mood and memory abilities.

To truly nourish yourself, and to obtain a clear, calm, and creative mind, you should aim to eat whole, real foods that have one ingredient—for example, apples, onions, mussels, almonds, and chicken. These foods contain more of the good stuff (vitamins, minerals, phytonutrients, and fiber) and less of the bad stuff (toxins). My goal in this book is to provide you with a practical and enticing tool: know what your body needs and why, and then fuel it via simple, efficient recipes.

Food on the Couch

When it comes to mental health, it's important to keep in mind that this is a complex area and everyone's situation is unique. But sometimes we make even the simplest elements too complex. Here is the straight truth: the human body and brain run on a core set of nutrients. The majority of people do not meet the daily requirement of many of these nutrients. If you become deficient in any of the key nutrients your brain and body need, you cannot function at your best. You may feel run-down, irritable, sluggish, and sad.

For many people, these are the long-term consequences of poor nutrition and lifestyle choices. Take Tommy, for example. Tommy never imagined he would see a psychiatrist. He had just graduated from college and was a hardworking, smart, and thoughtful young man. But he couldn't find a job after college, and he ended up moving back in with his mom and dad. He abandoned his fitness routine, his friends got busy with work and new girlfriends, and the structure of his life evaporated.

He was depressed when we met and had even pondered suicide. He had no job, no apartment, no girlfriend, and no hope. He slept all day and played video games late into the night. He started to blow up at his parents. He was irritable, went through mood swings, and became isolated.

Embarrassed by his situation, Tommy asked me if he was bipolar. He wasn't—he was malnourished. With each new patient comes a new food story, and Tommy's story was particularly vivid. I asked him to take a picture of everything he ate for three days, and the collection of pictures told a story of empty carbohydrates, missing fats, and a tribute to the color beige: bagels, breakfast cereal, pasta, pizza, hot dogs. When I joked that he should eat more colors, he sent a picture of colorful gummy bears.

But Tommy knew enough about nutrition to see the problem, commenting that he ate "like a twelve-year-old boy." As it turned out, he had always been interested in food, which helped facilitate his quest to feel better. First, he agreed to focus his schedule so that he was sleeping during the night and awake in time for breakfast every morning. One of the symptoms of depression is a lack of appetite, and lower food intake means fewer essential nutrients for the brain. Together we set some modest breakfast goals for him, and the first was to include more plants in his diet. With the help of a blender, Tommy started looking forward to his morning smoothie of fruits, greens, and nuts blended with yogurt and a bit of honey.

Pasta and carbs have a bad reputation, but together we were able to transform these dishes into something healthier. Tommy ate ravioli stuffed with Swiss chard and butternut squash. He started to use grass-fed beef for his Bolognese sauce and added some carrots. He'd never considered eating seafood, but eventually he tried linguini and clam sauce, with plenty of garlic. Pasta became a delivery vehicle for new foods and an opportunity to add more brain food to his diet.

As Tommy changed his food, he changed his brain and its nutritional profile. By adding in more plants and consuming fewer white carbs, Tommy increased the nutrient density of his diet and started feeding his microbiome, the trillions of bacteria in your gut that greatly influence your immune system and brain health. Adding in seafood meant supplying high concentrations of vitamin B_{12}, zinc, and the long-chained omega-3 fats—likely the three most critical brain nutrients. He also started receiving a supply of phytonutrients for the first time. These molecules protect our cells and turn on genes that promote our health. When I finally saw him grin one afternoon, it was like a rusty gear coming back to life.

Tommy soon started a new job at a gym and then began leading hikes for a local tour company. He even met a young woman and fell in love (really!). His battle against depression ended in a victory, and this success stayed with me. Food as an intervention helped Tommy on multiple levels, from the molecular to the psychological. Months after he left treatment, I wrote to check on him. His world had continued to expand socially and he was applying to graduate school. He wrote back, "I know one thing is true. If I don't eat right, I don't feel right." It seems such a simple truth: nothing can replace proper nourishment.

Unlike vitamin D and vitamin B_{12}, many of the 21 nutrients in this book are not included in routine blood analysis at the doctor's office. We don't check zinc levels or magnesium levels routinely. We don't measure the omega-3 fat content of your cells or check to see if your veins are coursing with flavanols. The only way to ensure you get enough nutrients is to eat the right foods. Working with Tommy cemented the idea that I should include a food assessment for every patient I evaluate. How could I properly treat my patients without knowing what they eat?

A few weeks later, a patient from my past returned to my couch. This young woman had been working abroad, and on her return to New York she found herself back in a rut. Her brain felt foggy and forgetful, which left her struggling at work. She was sad and cried easily, calling herself an emotional mess. She exercised intensely and was constantly hungry, and yet for all her efforts, she couldn't lose weight or feel better. She was single, miserable, and thirty pounds overweight, facing the daily onslaught of life in New York City. On top of all this, she was frequently sick with a cold or cough.

Our conversation turned to food and she told me she had stopped eating meat, seafood, and dairy for the last year, a choice she considered healthy and better for the planet. But then she lowered her voice and added, "But I have been craving meat every night. What's that about?"

I had a few ideas. Her diet was very low in iron and zinc, it contained no vitamin B_{12}, and she didn't eat a single milligram of the fat most important to human brain health: DHA, the long-chained omega-3 fat. These are four of the most valuable nutrients for brain health, and she was getting almost none of them from her diet. She had a few supplements she was supposed to take, including a multivitamin and iron prescribed by her doctor. But she found that these supplements had slipped to the back of her shelf, ignored and forgotten. Supplements are helpful to restore nutrient deficiencies, but for long-term health, nothing beats food.

Helping my patient eat meat and seafood in a way that felt right to her was a cornerstone of helping her get better. Seafood and meat are where you find the most absorbable form of all of the nutrients she was missing: vitamin B_{12}, long-chained omega-3 fats, zinc, and heme iron, a highly absorbable form found in meat and seafood.

Over time, she learned to eat complete, and her overall health and happiness began to improve. Today she is married and has a beautiful young son. She has lost weight, but more importantly she has energy, a brighter outlook, and a much better sense of focus and purpose.

These examples and many others have reinforced my belief that the best way to influence my patients' nutritional health is to help shape their everyday decisions about food. This seems to be the only method to ensure their brains are properly nourished. And a well-nourished brain functions better overall: it's more resilient in the face of stressors, it's more focused, and it provides a more stable mood. Evidence also shows that food is the largest factor within your control that can help preserve memory and decrease your risk of dementia as well as depression. With such far-reaching benefits for your brain and for your overall health, it's clear there is much to be gained by eating complete—eat right to feel right, and you have nothing to lose.

Nutrition Math

How many calories are in six oysters? I've asked this question of thousands of people around the country, to a wide variety of responses. One physician even guessed 875 calories.

The point here is that while we are regularly told to watch our calories, most of us have no idea how many calories are in the foods that we eat. When I first started paying attention to food, I realized I didn't know the calorie count of an egg or an apple. An oyster (10–20 calories) is even more exotic. Instead, we rely on a label to give us calorie counts, and this drives us to pick up packaged foods rather than whole foods.

But if we don't know much about calorie counts, we know even less about other important nutritional values—and these other values have great importance to our overall health. My focus with these recipes is to give you all of the nutritional numbers, so that you can see the simple truth of how food is medicine. This book does some serious nutrient counting for you, but at the end, I hope you'll forget all of the figures. They are here for guidance and reassurance, but the road to being a "Compleater" is paved with food, not numbers.

My goal, therefore, is not to inspire obsessive calorie or nutrient counting. If there is a mantra I try to instill in patients, it is to stop counting calories and instead keep track of certain nutrients of particular importance. This is easy when you choose to eat the foods that are the top sources of the essential 21 nutrients you need. And these foods form the foundation of each recipe in this book.

For example, I don't know how many

milligrams of omega-3 fats I eat each week. Instead, I know that I eat the best sources of these special fats three or four times per week: wild salmon, oysters, and maybe some anchovies in a kale Caesar salad. No one likes the idea of turning meals into math equations, and leaning too heavily on nutritional statistics can strip people of their most important asset when it comes to food: intuition.

Don't let all the brain science and obsessive nutrient counting mislead you—healthy food is pretty simple. Personally, I'm an easygoing cook and eater. In the summers, I like to grow food, pick it, and cook it up in a simple fashion. If you skip the growing and picking part, it is easier and less expensive to eat complete than ever before. We have an abundance of choice when it comes to fresh, healthy, affordable food.

My patients have been the main inspiration behind this approach to food. One of the harder parts of my job as a shrink is helping people change their ingrained habits and attitudes. Telling someone to eat more zinc is not helpful, as most folks don't know where to find zinc, other than in a multivitamin. Even if you know that oysters are high in zinc, raw oysters are a strange and slimy prescription for many people. A better solution is to give someone a recipe loaded with zinc, such as the grilled oyster tacos on page 252 or the shredded beef soup on page 201. Ta-da:

zinc is part of your diet, and you're one step closer to a completely nourished brain.

Your Brain Is Hungry

Over the last decade, medical research published in the top-tier medical journals—the *New England Journal of Medicine*, the *Journal of the American Medical Association*, and the *American Journal of Psychiatry*—has supported what common sense has told us for centuries: food choices have a huge impact on our risk of diseases, for everything ranging from heart disease and diabetes (which you probably knew) to the risk of depression and dementia (which many people are surprised to learn).

So what exactly does brain health have to do with food? It turns out, just about everything. Stop eating foods with iodine, and you won't be able to crack a smile—plus you'll slowly gain weight. Eat in way that depletes your stores of vitamin B_{12} or iron, and you'll notice you can't think as clearly. Your brain is in many ways an extension of your gut. Skip the foods that nourish your gut with healthy bacteria, and you can't get past that feeling of worry. Your brain is in control of it all, from your mood, energy level, and memory to your weight, appetite, and ability to sleep.

Brain cells are the hungriest in your body and, consequently, your brain uses more of the food you eat than any other organ. It makes up only 2 percent of your body weight, yet it burns around 420 calories a day. That is the equivalent of running four miles! So what does your brain do with all of those calories? A complex tangle of brain cells, fat, and cholesterol, your brain is coursing with electricity. The electrical rhythms within your brain are so strong that they can be measured with an Electroencephalogram (EEG), and we can see when they are not functioning properly (for example, when people have a seizure).

You can imagine that one hundred billion cells all generating a small bit of electricity create a high demand for fuel, and this explains why brain cells are your hungriest cells. And the need for so much cell activity is what determines the essential 21 nutrients. Many of the nutrients in the essential 21, such as vitamin B_1, are required to burn that fuel by turning sugars and fats into energy inside the cell. Others, such as vitamin C and several of the phytonutrients, help you deal with the waste. Much as in a woodstove or a car, burning fuel for the brain is an act of combustion that creates waste—and this waste needs to be cleaned up.

Nutrients such as vitamin E and omega-3 fats protect your brain directly. They eliminate free radicals and reduce inflammation. Others, such as the phytonutrient sulforaphane, help your brain by increasing the amount of enzymes in your liver that eliminate toxins, thereby coaxing your body into a natural state of increased detoxification (and this biological level of detox is far more important than a short, unsustainable regimen of rose petal water and cayenne).

Eating complete allows your very hungry brain cells to fuel and detox the brain—and leaves your brain and body to function at their very best as a result.

Brain Growth

By eating food containing concentrations of the essential 21 nutrients, you achieve more than simply providing the raw ingredients needed for brain function—you also send a signal to the brain to create new cells. A number of nutrients are now known to influence a process called neurogenesis, or the birth of new brain cells. This is a relatively new concept in medicine, as for decades we believed that brain cells could not regenerate and that the adult brain slowly lost brain cells over time. Today we know that the adult brain has the capacity to grow new brain cells, and that you can enhance this process by eating the right foods.

Molecules were discovered that trigger the growth of new brain cells, and they also happen to promote the health and resiliency of your existing brain cells. The most powerful of these is Brain Derived Neurotrophic Factor (BDNF), a hormone made by your cells. Low levels are strongly correlated with depression, but a number of nutrients in this book directly increase the expression of BDNF. While several genetic factors can influence BDNF and brain health, eating more of the nutrients that boost your levels is a great way to improve your health and decrease your risk of illness. The recipes in this book aim to maximize your intake of the nutrients known to have a positive impact on BDNF: omega-3 fats, zinc, magnesium, the flavonoid family of phytonutrients, and curcumin, found in the spice turmeric.

The biggest promise of this book is a shift in your brain chemistry. If your brain cells are bathed in the right nutrients, they will start to grow. If your adult brain has the capacity to continue growing, this provides a new frontier of possibility.

The Taste of Science

There are three main kinds of research that determine the nutrients and inform the recipes in this book. The first source is epidemiological studies. These are the studies of large populations that carefully track what people eat, control for confounding factors such as smoking or exercise, and then follow these individuals over a number of years to see what happens. They can tell us a great deal about correlations—for example, women who eat more fish during pregnancy have children who have 7.5 more verbal IQ points, showing a correlation between maternal fish consumption and offspring IQ.

It may sound far-fetched to some that changing what you eat can change your brain. But that's exactly what a 2015 study found. Researchers at the Australian National University followed 255 people over four years and assessed their diets. The subjects' brains were carefully measured with MRI brain scans at the beginning and end of the study. After four years, those who ate the most nutrient-dense foods had a left hippocampus that was 45 cubic millimeters bigger, which is about the size of a grain of rice and equal to millions of brain cells.This brain area is the center of our emotional regulation and learning. A bigger hippocampus means more brain cells in the area of the brain that helps dictate our overall happiness, giving you more brain power to understand your feelings and to learn.

Another compelling epidemiological study comes from researchers in Spain at the University of Las Palmas de Gran Canaria. Researchers tracked 10,094 university students over four years while assessing their diet and mental health. They found that the students who adhered most closely to the Mediterranean dietary pattern had a 42 percent reduced risk of depression during this period. This remarkable study has profound implications about how to decrease the burden of depression—by preventing it. If you don't suffer from depression, you may wonder how this applies to your life. We are all at risk for brain illnesses such as depression, just as we are all at risk for heart disease and cancer. However, unlike heart disease and cancer, mental illness strikes at earlier ages, most often during the early and middle adult years, and it is the top cause of disability worldwide. What we cook for our family and friends is one of our most powerful weapons to help prevent mental illness.

A number of studies have replicated this result and consistently show that populations who eat the foods in this book have lower rates of depression and dementia, two illnesses that rob us of our human potential. The brain is both marvelous and fragile at the same time. From these population studies, we see the potential that dietary changes have in dictating brain health. It is not a coincidence that the nutrient-dense foods that form the core of *Eat Complete* are also the stars of the Mediterranean diet and other traditional diets: fresh vegetables, leafy greens, nuts, olive oil, seafood, and grass-fed meat and dairy.

Population studies also look at how certain nutrients, such as the amount of omega-3 fats in one's diet, correlate with the risk of certain illnesses. A number of studies show clear evidence that the B vitamins, the omega-3 fats, zinc, iron, and a number of plant-based phytonutrients are negatively correlated with the rate at which the human brain shrinks, meaning that—for example—a higher level of vitamin B_{12} in your blood is positively correlated with having more brain cells and more connections between cells. Studies like this make me crave a plate of *pasta vongole*, as clams are the top source of vitamin B_{12}.

To prove causation—that changing what you eat can change your brain health for the better and shift the trajectory of your life—researchers employ controlled, randomized trials in which individuals are given an intervention. This is the second main source of research that informs this book. While such trials are the gold standard of proof in medicine, these studies are challenging; getting people to adhere to a specific diet over months if not years is difficult and very expensive to study. However, a recent trial found that counseling elderly depressive patients about food reduced their depression symptoms by half. Another trial gave nuts to one group of patients and compared them with a group of patients given olive oil instead. After two years, the group that received the nuts were protected against severely low levels of brain growth factor BDNF.

Other clinical trials have used nutrients such as the omega-3 fats, zinc, and B vitamins in supplement form in the treatment of disorders: for instance, one trial showed fish oil to be equal to Prozac in the treatment of depression. In 2015, the first trial of a probiotic to treat depression was completed with positive results. The data has been so compelling that multiple clinical trials are under way around the world to study the treatment of depression with a traditional Mediterranean-style diet.

Finally, there is the data that comes from the study of how certain molecules interact with our DNA. Studies in test tubes and petri dishes do not give us conclusive evidence, but they can show us the elegant biological mechanisms of the molecules in your food. It's compelling to learn that vitamin K is needed to construct sphingolipids, the complex fat cells in your brain; or that lycopene cells from tomatoes can be found in brain cells after a meal. Omega-3 fats bind to our DNA and trigger the production of a brain growth factor, which seems to be a clear sign that we should eat foods that contain these fats.

All of this data guides us towards foods and food rules that are not necessarily considered the standard fare of healthy eaters. For example, by asking you to focus on eating specific brain nutrients, I am thereby recommending a diet that contains both fats and cholesterol. This challenges a basic tenet that many eaters live by: that we should eliminate fat and cholesterol from our diets. But a careful considation of the data reveals that dietary cholesterol has no clear impact on health or health outcomes and little effect on the cholesterol levels that your doctor checks. That's why the new 2015 Dietary Recommendations for Americans by the USDA eliminated cholesterol as a "nutrient of concern for overconsumption." And a careful reading of the scientific literature, including a meta-analysis of twenty-one published research trials by Harvard University researcher Patty Siri-Tarino, PhD, reveals that our obsession with eliminating fats and saturated fats is also misguided. Further refutation of the case against fat and cholesterol has been undertaken by journalist Gary Taubes in his book *Good Calories, Bad Calories*, along with Nina Teicholz's *The Big Fat Surpise* and in the blogs of physicians such as Emily Deans, MD; Peter Attia, MD; and Robert Lustig, MD. (Dr. Attia's nine-part blog post, "The Straight Dope on Cholesterol," deserves special mention.) While we were taught that fat and cholesterol are unhealthy, the science now shows that they should not be at the top of your list of concerns about food, if on the list at all.

Health, wellness, and food advice is often polarized and extreme, which is a troubling pattern given that our understanding of food and wellness continues to evolve. When health and wellness experts are honest and helpful, there is more shrugging and encouragement, and a lot less dogma and judgment. After all, we should be in service of your health, not of our message. This problematic approach to health and wellness messaging is what drove me to focus on these 21 nutrients. People will continue to debate the health merits of certain fats, butter, eggs, and meat, but there is no debate about the pressing daily need for a diet rich in omega-3 fats, vitamin B_{12}, zinc, magnesium, and the other nutrients on which this book focuses.

Ultimately, it's the science of food that matters. Many people I meet are confused about what constitutes a healthy meal. Some are misled by the supplement industry, some by the big marketing budgets of the large food companies that make cheap, packaged foods, and even more by the steady stream of contradictory health headlines in the news. Stop listening to all the noise and headlines. Stop wasting your money on supplements. Stop believing claims on labels.

Your health is in your control. You want to feel better, and feel good about what you eat? Eat complete and you will.

Eat Complete Tips

It takes more than just nutrients to transform your health. You also need to connect with yourself and your food: how you eat, with whom you eat, and where you buy your food are factors that you need to consider to truly eat complete. It's not that a dinner of wild salmon, quinoa, and kale scarfed down in front of the TV is horrible, but consciously emphasizing your connection to your food and your food system yields great health benefits. In addition, your body must be in a relaxed state to be able to optimally digest and absorb the nutrients from your food.

The following suggestions are designed to help increase your enjoyment of the food you eat, as well as promote better digestion:

Eat Mindfully

Mindfulness means being present moment to moment. Eating complete works best if you are fully present with your food. It is beneficial to your digestion if you slow down before you eat, and the best way to accomplish this is to practice mindfulness. Luckily, this is easy to do.

Before you eat anything, try taking a deep breath. Inhale fully through your nose and then slowly exhale with your mouth, through pursed lips. Try to clear your mind while doing this. Then use all of your senses to appreciate your food. Appreciate the colors on your plate and the aroma of the meal. Appreciate your company if you have it.

Slowing down also helps ensure better digestion. When you create time for a meal to hit your senses, the appearance and smell and first tastes will increase your production of saliva and other digestive enzymes, all of which help your body break down the food and release its nutrients.

One breath. One bite at a time. Be mindful of your food.

Foster an Attitude of Gratitude

In our house, we try to start meals with a moment of silence so that we can pause to appreciate our food. We live in a world of excess stress and distraction, and that's probably not going to change for most of us. But mealtimes can be insulated from all this stress by the simple act of appreciating the food in front of you. For some, this is a spiritual moment giving thanks to the power in the universe that brought the food to your table. For others, it is just a simple thanks. Millions of people on our planet go hungry every day. Be thankful you are not one of them. Appreciate those who toiled to grow your food and the many steps involved in getting it onto the plate in front of you.

Chew

To release the nutrients bound up within your food, you need to use all the digestive power you have. Most digestion is involuntary, a miracle of breaking down and extracting nutrients from food. You don't have to focus on absorbing iron or B_{12}, for example—it just happens automatically. Chewing is the one part of digestion over which you have control. There is no optimal number, but try starting with ten chews per bite. To most people, this feels like a lot, but more chewing breaks down the components of your food and mixes it with salivary enzymes. Plus, extra chewing slows down your eating and prevents you from scarfing down everything on your plate.

No Screens at the Table

You have plenty of time for screen addiction. After you snap a picture of your food and post it to social media (perhaps tagging it #eatcomplete), turn off your ringer and put away your phone. If your screen addiction is getting out of control, put your phone in another room. Turn off the TV as well, even if it is in another room. Watching shows or movies during meals is the epitome of mindless eating and a sure path to weight gain and unhappiness.

Why Not Just Take a Multivitamin?

The first vitamin was isolated in 1912. Just over 100 years later, taking supplements has become part of everyday modern life—an "insurance policy" for missing nutrients in our diet. Mulitvitamins and other supplements are a simple and effective way to improve the vitamin and mineral status of patients who suffer from some medical conditions. For example, people with illnesses such as pernicious anemia can't absorb vitamin B_{12} and require a supplement. Many people face a vitamin D deficiency and in the winter need a vitamin D supplement to bring their levels up to normal. For most people, however, the insurance policy of a daily multivitamin is a hollow promise.

It may technically be possible to survive on a diet of a multivitamin, sugar, water, soy protein powder, a shot of essential oils, and a few scoops of Metamucil for fiber. But it's a slippery slope when we remove ourselves and our nutritional needs from the food cycle and our knowledge of food is lost. When that happens, one can easily adopt the attitude that it doesn't matter if you eat healthily or not, because of your multivitamin insurance policy.

But multivitamins can't compare to the power of food. First, there is an absorption issue. For example, cation minerals such as calcium, magnesium, and iron compete for transporters in the gut and block one another's absorption. Another issue is that the phytonutrients in plants aren't found in most multivitamins. Many supplements use blends of dehydrated food concentrates, though these certainly are not equivalent to the compounds found in plants. Generally, supplements come in concentrations and forms not found in nature. There is also the reductionist notion that if some amount enhances our health, a larger quantity gives us even better health. For example, while resveratrol is an interesting molecule found in grapes and wine that enhances expression of the SIRT genes (which slow aging in animal models), this does not mean that a supplement containing the resveratrol equivalent to 500 bottles of wine promotes health.

Then there is the risk of supplements. Unfortunately, many people trust the supplement industry because they are suspicious of pharmaceutical companies and supplements are supposed to be "natural." But "Big Pharma" must rigorously test its medicines and monitor them for safety, whereas the supplement industry does not go through the same rules and regulations. A quick glance at the FDA safety warning and recall list reveals the truth. Many supplements are contaminated with heavy metals such as lead and cadmium, contain adulterants that could trigger allergies, and often contain pharmaceutical drugs (such as natural sleeping pills that contain drug analogs of Valium, or energy supplements that contain ephedrine—both of which are powerful medications with their own risks).

Finally, no one ever sat down and savored a meal of vitamins and supplement shakes. Reducing food to just a set of nutrients leaves out the many ways that food connects us to ourselves, to one another, and to our food system. Our knowledge of nutrition should lead us back to the dinner table, not to the supplement aisle.

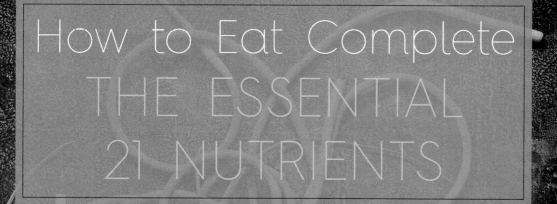

How to Eat Complete

THE ESSENTIAL
21 NUTRIENTS

B oth common sense and modern science tell us food choices present the greatest opportunity to influence your health. And the effects of eating nutrient-dense foods are quickly apparent: a boost in energy, better sleep, a more stable mood, and improved focus. Other benefits, such as better memory as you age, are longer term.

But even with your health on the line and ample motivation, many people still struggle with the basic question. *How do you eat complete?*

Eat Complete offers a simple solution: focus on eating the most concentrated sources of the most important nutrients for your brain. In this chapter, we'll review each of the 21 nutrients and why they made the list (hint: science). We'll highlight how these nutrients build and fuel the brain. You will also learn about challenges and tricks to eating complete (for example, how to ensure the greatest absorption). Most importantly, you will learn the top food sources of these nutrients—meaning which foods have the highest nutrient content. These foods will be the building blocks of the recipes in this book.

This chapter will also familiarize you with the nutrients you will see throughout the book and will serve as a reference for you going forward. Not sure why there are cashews in your smoothie and clams on your pizza? Can't remember why you should be so crazy for vitamin B_{12} and omega-3 fats? Informed eaters make the best choices. I hope you will use the following information both as a reference and as motivation—and most importantly, use it to help you fuel your brain.

The Rules of Kale

There are three rules that can help you spot an important brain food, and kale actually provides a great framework for these three lessons. Let's call them the Rules of Kale. The first rule is **Nutrient Density**, which focuses on eating with efficiency, so that every calorie brings a bevy of nutrients. The foods with the highest concentration of nutrients should be the foundation of your diet.

The second rule is that foods need **Culinary Flexibility**, so that eaters aren't bored by the same thing and can instead create diverse feasts with a few foods. Bring some kale to my house and you could find yourself eating kale and eggs, a kale smoothie, or a kale salad. We might make some kale pesto, or even a "kalejito." Kale is incredibly versatile and can be added to almost any dish to make it healthier.

The third rule is **Local Access**, which encourages people to connect to their food supply, eat with a smaller footprint, and eat seasonal food. Access also means that the food is affordable and available, something that can be a challenge. Leafy greens form the base of the food supply—they grow almost everywhere, and they are affordable for nearly everyone. Given the spread of farmers' markets nationally (by last count we have 8,144 in the United States), along with many state programs that double the value of food stamps at farmers' markets, Americans' access to fresh, local, nutrient-dense produce is increasing.

Following these three rules and eating a diet based on foods with the highest concentrations of the essential 21 helps ensure that your brain is nourished—and it's easy and affordable to do so.

Compleater Principles

As my quest for the 21 nutrients and where to find them unfolded, several themes emerged that apply to this pattern of eating complete. I've grouped them here into a set of principles that will help guide you in your journey to becoming a "Compleater":

- Plant Based
- Complex Carbohydrates
- Sensible Seafood
- Microbiome Cultivation
- Whole and Fermented Grains
- Grass-Fed Meat, Dairy, and Eggs
- Natural Colors and Flavors
- Organic When Possible

Plant Based

Eating more of the right plants increases the nutrient density of your diet, as you get more nutrients per calorie from things such as leafy greens and beans than you do from meat. This is one of the reasons that vegetarians have healthier weights. All plant foods are mostly water, which helps you stay naturally hydrated. Plants are also chock-full of phytonutrients like carotenoids and flavanols, which are magic molecules that do much more in your body than simply act as antioxidants (see phytonutrients on page 62). Getting a variety of phytonutrients by "eating the rainbow" of plants helps lower inflammation, promote a healthy gut, and turn on genes that fight disease. You also ensure that the bacteria in your microbiome are getting their favorite food—fiber. In addition, plants are the only good source of vitamin C, which humans can't make themselves. And along with the health benefits, eating more plants is easy on your budget and makes you a better environmental citizen. Increasing your intake of plant-based proteins such as lentils and beans is an important step in shifting your eating patterns to include more plants.

Complex Carbohydrates

Complex carbohydrates, such as those in legumes, whole grains, and nuts, are a great fuel for human health. But the carbs in many diets are simple sugars and refined carbohydrates, which are the top drivers of illness, weight gain, and brain drain. These go by hundreds of names: corn syrup solids, organic cane sugar, dextrose, crystalline fructose, invert sugar, coconut sugar, apple juice concentrate, potato starch, rice flour, enriched bleached brominated flour, and refined grains of all kinds. A key to understanding your health comes from understanding glucose. This simple sugar is the main sugar operating in your blood and the main fuel of the brain. It is the primary sugar found in all plants, as it is the building block of both starch and fiber. Humans are wired to seek simple sugars and sweet tastes because these signal safe calories. But this instinct has been hijacked by modern food, leading to a steady diet of simple sugar and empty calories that contain none of the essential 21 nutrients. By eating whole foods and thus primarily complex carbohydrates such as the sugars found in lentils, amaranth, and avocados, you will have a fuel source that digests more slowly, contains more nutrients, and feeds your microbiome. This doesn't mean no dessert. Instead, it means ensuring that every bite, even dessert, has some of the nutrients you need.

Sensible Seafood

The human brain evolved along the coastlines and shorelines for good reason. Seafood contains the most essential minerals, vitamins, and fats for brain function—namely, the long-chained omega-3 fats, zinc, iron, vitamin B_{12}, and iodine. The largest creation of energy on the planet likely happens in the ocean via algae and phytoplankton, and these tiny creatures are the origin of the long-chained omega-3 fats that are concentrated in the fish and other seafood that eat them. Bivalves, mussels, clams, oysters, and scallops are top sources of vitamin B_{12}. Generally, wild-caught seafood is best for eating complete because farmed seafood has a different nutrient profile due to differences in the animals' diet and environment.

Microbiome Cultivation

From fighting bacteria to prescribing bacteria, the medical world is just beginning to understand the important role played by the many residents of your gut. A collection of trillions of bacteria, called the microbiome, resides there. This might seem out of place in a cookbook, but the bacteria in your gastrointestinal system are necessary companions to your health. They also possess a number of powers, such as the ability to break down fibers. Your human cells hold a measly 23,000 genes, but the bacteria in your microbiome collectively have more than two million genes.

The makeup of your microbiome is based on the foods you eat. Eating more plants for a few days is enough to shift and alter the types of bacteria that predominate in your gut. Adding fermented foods to your diet, such as yogurt and kefir, provides many species of *Lactobacillus* and *Bifidobacter* bacteria, two families of bacteria that seem to promote health. Every culture around the globe has a set of fermented foods in its diet, and for good reason. Along with live bacterial cultures that populate the gut, the fermentation process helps digest and transform foods, creating unique forms of vitamins such as vitamin K_2.

Whole and Fermented Grains

This book is 99 percent gluten-free, to help shake things up in your approach to grains. A single grain dominates modern diets: wheat. While nutrient dense, it is primarily eaten as refined flour stripped of its nutrients and phytonutrients. Between 1 and 2 percent of people have celiac disease, an autoimmune condition in which wheat is toxic. An additional small percentage of people, perhaps 5 to 6 percent in the United States, are intolerant of wheat. Most people do not have an issue digesting gluten and I don't believe that gluten is toxic for everyone. But I made this book mainly gluten-free for two reasons. The first is that most eaters have no problem getting plenty of wheat and gluten in their diet—both are ubiquitous in modern food. Extra gluten is added to most baked goods, to soy sauce, and even to meats, like ham.

There's now an emerging connection between unhealthy guts, overexposure to gluten, and a host of health and mental health conditions. Second, we have some nonceliac gluten intolerance in our house, and I know it is tough for families like ours to stay clear of gluten. Instead of including gluten-containing grains in this book, I've included some gluten-free grain options, all of which are nutrient dense and more fun in the kitchen—such as quinoa, which has six times more magnesium compared with wheat and 25 percent more iron. Fermenting flour with sourdough starter is another great option, a traditional preparation that increases flour's nutritional value and makes grains more digestible. Grains are a key part of the global food supply, and exploring other grain options provides new opportunities in the kitchen—mixing things up is the way to start making dietary changes.

Sourdough

Fermentation happens naturally. Yeast and bacteria work together to digest sugars and starches, which makes the nutrients more digestible. The sourness of sourdough comes from the acids made by this fermentation. A sourdough starter is a living colony that is kept in the refrigerator and requires regular care and feeding. The starter makes it easy to produce dough for bread or batter for pancakes or waffles. You can make your own starter with flour, water, and airborne yeast; get a starter from a fermentation-savvy friend; or buy a commercial sourdough starter. Fermenting can greatly reduce the amount of gluten, though readers with true celiac disease should use gluten-free flours. *The Art of Fermentation* by Sandor Katz is a great guide to learning this ancient, simple craft.

Grass-Fed Meat, Dairy, and Eggs

Few foods polarize eaters like meat and the debate about its effect on health. Ninety-nine percent of people eat meat or some animal product such as dairy. Improving the quality, and for most people decreasing the quantity, of this meat is one of the key messages I hope to impart. The average American eats over 250 pounds of meat per year, an amount associated with obesity, heart disease, dementia, and cancer—not to mention the huge environmental costs. If eating plants and seafood provides you with the most critical of the 21 nutrients, is there any reason to include meat, dairy, and eggs?

If meat, dairy, and eggs are done right, they offer a nutrient-dense, healthy, sustainable food choice. Meat, dairy, and eggs all provide a complete protein, one with all nine essential amino acids. Though this is possible to achieve by combining plants, such as beans and rice, plants are much lower in protein. The iron in meat is a more highly absorbable form of iron called heme iron, which is notable for those struggling with iron deficiency anemia. Meat, dairy, and eggs also all contain vitamin B_{12}, but to do these foods right means they must come from a pasture-raised animal, ideally from a farm near you. Raising animals in pastures creates meat, dairy, and eggs with more nutrient density, and also a more diverse mix of nutrients. For example, pasture-raised meat and dairy contain much more conjugated linoleic acid (CLA). This fat appears to help the body build muscle and decrease fat storage. Researchers call it a "body composition modulator." Grass-fed meat and dairy contain more CLA compared with conventionally raised meat, and they also contain small amounts of the long-chained omega-3 fats EPA and DHA, which are central to brain health. For people who don't eat seafood, this is one of the few food sources of these fats. Meat from grass-fed animals also has higher concentrations of provitamin A carotenoids (which can be seen in the yellow color of the fat) and vitamin E, two antioxidants that cool inflammation. And because this meat contains less fat, it also has fewer calories. Just switching to grass-fed beef would save

most eaters between 15,000 and 20,000 calories per year.[*]

Some eaters are concerned about reports that meat can increase the risk of cancer. In 2015, the World Health Organization issued a statement that a high intake of processed meat and red meat (meaning near-daily consumption) is linked with a slight increase in cancer risk. It is important to understand that this kind of study does not mean meat causes cancer. However, high intakes of red meat and highly processed meat do present a number of health and environmental problems. My aim with the meat recommendations in this book is to help you enjoy meat if that is your preference, without concerns about future health issues.

Meat is a problem for the majority of eaters I see. There is a reliance on convenient, cheap meats such as ham, chicken breasts, and turkey bacon. There is also a lack of diversity in terms of which parts of the animal are consumed—meaning many of the most nutrient-dense parts of the animal, such as liver, other organ meats, and marrow, are wasted. Another common issue comes from meat products such as chicken tenders, hot pockets, and breaded cutlets, which don't provide much benefit

---

[*] I first saw a calculation like this on Jo Robinson's *Eat Wild* blog (www.eatwild.com/healthbenefits .htm).

from the meat, but do add sugar, refined carbohydrates, and empty calories to diets. Instead, if you choose nonprocessed, all grass-fed meat, and explore some high-value, high-flavor cuts such as beef shanks and liver, you will get more nutrients for fewer calories all while exploring a new, healthier relationship with meat.

Dairy can cause problems for some people, but much of the dairy included in this book is fermented. This eliminates much of the sugar lactose, which is what causes bloating and gas for people with lactose intolerance, and it also breaks down the dairy proteins, which can make dairy tolerable for people with mild dairy sensitivity.

Eggs possess the perfect protein by which all other proteins are measured. In fact, every nutrient a brain cell needs can be found in an egg. They are also the top source of choline, a vitamin closely related to B vitamins, and the most recent addition by the Institute of Medicine to the list of dietary essential nutrients. Eggs are low calorie, nutrient dense, and filling, but they've been caught in controversies about heart health because they are high in cholesterol. The cholesterol profile your doctor tests has very little to do with the amount of cholesterol you eat, though. And in fact, much of the cholesterol in an egg isn't even absorbed. As the science of blood cholesterol, diet, and heart disease has evolved, it has become clear that sugars, refined carbohydrates, and trans fats are more responsible for heart disease than cholesterol and eggs. The 2015 Dietary Guidelines for Americans reflect this, as the daily limit on dietary cholesteral was removed. Remember, one of the main tasks of your body is to make cholesterol—primarily in your liver, but also in your brain. So don't fear cholesterol, as all of your cells, hormones, and even vitamin D are made from it. For most of us, eggs are great to eat as a regular part of our diet.

Getting meat, dairy, and eggs that are produced without the use of antibiotics is important for public health. Eighty percent of antibiotics in the United States are used on livestock, not because the animals are sick, but because antibiotics promote growth. This overuse has led to an epidemic of antibiotic-resistant infections as bacteria with genes for resistance survive and multiply. One reason animals get sick is because they are confined. Another is that ruminants such as cows are meant to eat grass, not grains, which make the animals more prone to illness. Meat, dairy, and eggs from grass-fed animals is more nutritious and are better for our food chain overall.

Natural Colors and Flavors

Your sense of taste and smell are your brain's compass for food. Your brain and gut work in concert to decode this information, and color and flavor are key parts of the code. That's why eating fake foods with artificial colors and flavors is essentially lying to your brain.

The flavors and colors made in laboratories by food scientists are designed to hijack your senses, which is why we all struggle to eat just one potato chip or one cookie. The good news is that the recipes in this book are designed to satisfy. Even if you have been eating a lot of processed foods, the natural foods used here will provide both subtle and potent flavors. It takes several weeks to fully recover from a steady diet of highly processed foods, but luckily your sense of taste is highly sensitive and your set point for tastes is easily changed.

Finally, don't be fooled by the lure of no-calorie sweeteners. Studies show that people end up adding on these calories in other ways, because anything sweet still causes your body to respond as if you are eating sugars by releasing some insulin. Since food provides information to our bodies, it's best not to lie to our brains with fake colors or flavors.

Organic When Possible

I prefer to buy and grow organic food, but it isn't always possible to eat organic— particularly because the price is so often out of reach. Though the health benefits of eating organic food are difficult to prove,

most pesticides are made up of neurotoxins that kill brain cells, and I avoid these whenever possible out of common sense.

Certain foods require the extra effort (and cost) to buy the organic version. When you eat the skin of a food—think apples and berries versus a banana—organic matters even more. For leafy greens such as kale and mustard greens, you should choose organic. Choosing organic produce often steers us towards eating more seasonally, which is an easy way to ensure diversity in your diet and a quick cure for food boredom. If you are on a tight budget, freezing and canning during peak season offers great value.

Organic foods (particularly the fruits and vegetables) also usually contain more nutrients and more phytonutrients, as organic plants must defend themselves from pests and use phytonutrients to do so.

Some small farmers at your local farmers' market might use few to no chemicals, even if they are not certified organic. I encourage you to engage your local farmers about their practices.

The Essential 21

The word *essential* has a special meaning in medicine. Essential nutrients are typically ones you must eat because your body cannot produce them. For example, most mammals make vitamin C—but because humans cannot make it, we must consume it. Without a single essential nutrient, your health fails.

A few of the nutrients we will cover are not traditional "essential" nutrients. For example, the long-chained omega-3 fats EPA and DHA can be produced in the body, but health outcomes are better when we eat more of these fats in our diet. Thus, for the purposes of this book, you can think of this list as the essential 21 nutrients needed to transform your health through food. This means that there is strong evidence that these nutrients need to be part of our conversation about optimal health.

To eat complete, we seek those foods with the highest concentration of the essential 21 nutrients and the least number of calories. These nutrients were selected based on the latest science of how nutrients work in the brain and the increasing research that connects your dietary pattern to your brain function. The basic take-home message of the growing body of evidence is that eating nutrient-dense brain food can protect you from illnesses such as depression and dementia, and it can keep your brain bigger as you age compared with the brains of people who eat a "Western" diet (a.k.a. the SAD, Standard American Diet; or the MAD, Modern American Diet).

All of the essential 21 have known mechanisms for how they influence your health on the cellular level, and this is also supported by population studies and clinical trials. For example, a meta-analysis of high-quality studies found that low zinc levels are strongly correlated with depression, and that trials with zinc supplementation have shown positive effects on brain health. As it turns out, zinc is a critical factor in your body's defense system and thus key to feeling your best—but about half of the United States population does not meet the daily requirement for zinc.

This brings us to another important point. All of the essential 21 are also frequently lacking in most Western diets according to the daily nutrient requirement guidelines. In the United States and Canada, nutritional requirements called Dietary Reference Intakes are set by the Institute of Medicine's Food and Nutrition Board. This group of scientists reviews all of the research to best establish how much of a nutrient the average person needs to prevent deficiency in 95 percent of the population. This is called the Recommended Daily Allowance (RDA). The comprehensive literature review for each nutrient put forth by the Food and Nutrition Board has served as a primary resource for this book and is available free online for those of you who want to dig deeper.

Some nutrients do not have an RDA. When there is not enough science to determine an RDA, the Food and Nutrition Board establishes a level of Adequate Intake (AI). The amounts needed of different nutrients vary greatly, but the standard metrics for most macronutrients such as fats, proteins, and carbs are in terms of grams (g). Most vitamins and minerals are listed in milligrams (mg) and micrograms (mcg), respectively 1/1000 of a gram and 1/10,000 of a gram. So while you might require at least 2,000 milligrams or 2 grams of potassium a day, you require just 55 micrograms of selenium, which is .055 milligram or .000055 gram—just a dash.

THE ESSENTIAL 21

7 FOR FOUNDATION

1. Omega-3 Fats
2. Zinc
3. Vitamin B_{12}
4. Magnesium
5. Vitamin B_9
6. Good Bugs: Prebiotics and Probiotics
7. Complete Proteins

7 FOR PROTECTION

1. Vitamin E
2. Vitamin K
3. Vitamin A and Carotenoids
4. Phytonutrients: The Polyphenols
5. Monounsaturated Fats (MUFAs)
6. Vitamin D
7. Selenium

7 FOR IGNITION

1. Iron
2. Vitamin B_1
3. Choline
4. Calcium
5. Potassium
6. Iodine
7. Vitamin C

The nutrients are divided into three groups. In the first group, we focus on nutrients that are the foundation of brain health. These are the building blocks of a healthy, happy human brain and body. Once you have built a better brain, the second group of nutrients is focused on protecting it. These molecules eliminate free radicals (the waste), decrease inflammation, and keep our cellular machinery in tip-top shape. Included in the third group are nutrients most involved in energy production, as the brain has such a high metabolic rate. These nutrients both make cellular energy and also deal with the waste. Some of these nutrients could span all three categories, as they play many roles, but for our purposes we'll focus on the "ignition" properties involved in energy production.

My hope is that the information that follows will both motivate and help you to get more of the essential 21 in your diet. For each of these nutrients, we'll cover a bit about what it does in your body and brain. Many are involved in the same critical body processes: the creation and copying of DNA that are required every time a cell divides, the regulation of inflammation, and, of course, the growth of new brain cells and brain connections.

I have also listed how much you need of each nutrient according to the Dietary Reference Intake (DRI) of the Institute of Medicine. I've included the top food sources and also calculated the top recipes for each nutrient. To note, the percentages listed for the recipes are based on the daily need of women aged thirty-one to fifty. Generally, men's RDAs are a bit higher, and child and infant rates are much lower. For most nutrients, pregnancy and lactation increase demand. I've also included any important illnesses or factors that increase the risk of deficiency, as well as tips for absorption and cooking.

When you look at the listed rates of dietary insufficiency, the scope of our nation's nutrition problem is crystal clear. This is the percentage of Americans who *on average* don't meet the RDA of a given nutrient. This number was calculated using USDA data, recent epidemiology studies, and the National Health and Nutrition Examination Survey (NHANES), a project by the Centers for Disease Control (CDC) that assesses the nutritional status of the US population.

7 FOR FOUNDATION

Fats

Fats serve our body in three ways: as an energy source, as the building blocks of our cells, and as the precursors for signals that regulate brain growth, inflammation, hunger, and sugar. Your brain is mainly fat and so is your endocrine system, the part of your body that produces hormones such as insulin, cortisol, testosterone, and leptin, the hormones that regulate mood, energy metabolism, and growth. The mix of fats in our diets can be organized by their chemical structures: polyunsaturated, monounsaturated, and saturated. One goal for you as an eater is to have a more nuanced and informed view of fat. After all, you have more than 560 different kinds of fat in your blood!

While health messaging has focused on lowering fat and decreasing saturated fats in your diet, the actual risks associated with saturated fats are low. More importantly, some of the healthiest, longest-lived people on the planet eat a diet that is between 30 and 40 percent fat. Actually, the most dangerous fat in food is the one humans added to our food supply: *industrial trans fats.*

The *Eat Complete* goal regarding fats is to increase your intake of fats most associated with better health outcomes, namely monounsaturated fats and polyunsaturated fats, and to seek a better balance of the long-chained polyunsaturated fats by eating more omega-3 fats and fewer omega-6 fats. By following the recipes in this book, you won't eat anything that contains partially hydrogenated oils—meaning there are no industrial trans fats, which are estimated by Harvard University to cause 100,000 heart attacks per year and increase the risk of depression by 42 percent.

Omega-3 Fats

Omega-3 fats are also called polyunsaturated fats or PUFAs. They are the longest and most complex fats that you eat, and they play a variety of important roles in your brain: they serve as the building blocks of cell membranes, they stimulate the production of important brain growth factors, and they also directly regulate inflammation (among other things).

Omega-3 fats are essential, and you must eat them because your body cannot produce them. I use the phrase "one if by land, two if by sea" to remember that you get one omega-3 fat, ALA, from plant-based sources such as greens, flaxseeds, and chia seeds, and you get two, DHA and EPA, from seafood sources. But not all omega-3s are created equal, and an improvement of the omega-3 levels in your cells requires the longer forms found mainly in seafood. Just as important, you also need to balance omega-6 fats, which are more inflammatory, by eliminating vegetable oils like soy and sunflower oils.

Human brains, particularly growing human brains, are positively influenced by getting more of these fats. Researchers who study the evolution of the human brain note that the increased consumption of seafood led to a doubling of humanoid brain size in our ancestors. In the present day, studies of fish intake show that pregnant women who eat more fish and have higher levels of long-chained omega-3 fats have offspring with higher verbal IQs. While all forms of omega-3s are correlated with health and mental health benefits, the longer-chained kinds seem to impart the most benefit. These longer-chained forms are the ones used in clinical trials to treat and prevent depression, dementia, and heart disease.

In 2014, the USDA and the Environmental Protection Agency (EPA) drafted a statement reminding women to eat seafood two to three times per week, highlighting the importance of this food to brain development. It is critical, however, to choose fish that are high in omega-3 fats and low in mercury and other toxins by choosing smaller fish and bivalves and avoiding large predator fish. Have caution with farmed fish, as they can contain higher amounts of omega-6 fats from being raised on grain-based animal feed, and seek guidance on fish from local rivers and lakes, as contamination is unfortunately common.

ALPHA-LINOLENIC ACID (ALA) is the simplest and shortest of the omega-3 fats, and the most abundant fat on the planet. ALA is found in the leaves of plants, which use this special fatty acid to convert sunlight into energy. It is the major fat found in kale, Brussels sprouts, and broccoli, and it is especially concentrated in flaxseeds, purslane, and walnuts. You'll also find ALA in eggs and meat from pasture-raised animals.

Your body can convert some ALA into the longer-chained EPA and then DHA, but the conversion rate is quite low and it decreases as you age. People who do not eat long-chained omega-3 fats have lower levels in their cell membranes, which is why seafood is a recommended source of the omega-3s (see below for more). That said, ALA is a good fat with a number of health benefits.

AMOUNT YOU SHOULD EAT PER DAY: Women: 1.1g / Men: 1.6g

TOP 5 RECIPES FOR ALA
1. Sourdough Blueberry Pancakes = 252% (see page 130)
2. Mixed Nut–Cardamom Baklava Bites = 239% (see page 278)
3. Double-Green Summer Fritters = 157% (see page 182)
4. Baked Flaxseed Crab Cakes = 155% (see page 254)
5. Flourless Chocolate-Almond Cake = 150% (see page 279)

EICOSAPENTAENOIC ACID (EPA) plays a critical role in reducing inflammation. EPA is used by your body to make potent anti-inflammatory compounds that keep blood vessels relaxed and prevent blood clots. The more EPA there is in your diet, the lower the concentration of pro-inflammatory omega-6 fats in your cells. Your body can make EPA from ALA, but not very efficiently, which is why you need it in your diet. Low EPA is linked to depression, suicide, diabetes, and heart disease. EPA is found in fatty fish such as sardines, salmon, and mackerel; shellfish such as shrimp, oysters, and clams; and grass-fed mammals such as beef cattle, bison, sheep, and goats.

DOCOSAHEXAENOIC ACID (DHA) is the most abundant omega-3 fat in your brain and is highly concentrated in synapses, which are how brain cells connect to one another. Cells with more omega-3s in the membrane are more flexible, and this promotes better functioning. Along with its role as a fundamental building block of brain cells, DHA is also used to make potent hormones called neuroprotectins and resolvins, which combat inflammation and keep brain cells alive by blocking the signals that cause cell death. You need to eat several grams of DHA per week to maintain optimal concentrations in your tissues. Most countries have a daily recommendation of around 500mg per day for EPA and DHA combined—unlike the United States, which currently has no specific guidance on the long-chained PUFAs. Low levels of DHA are associated with depression, bipolar disorder, ADHD, and Alzheimer's disease. The most concentrated source of DHA is in cold-water fatty fish such as salmon, mackerel, and sardines. Vegetarians can get DHA from certain algae in supplement form as well.

AMOUNT YOU SHOULD EAT PER DAY: 500mg for women and men*

INSUFFICIENT DIETARY INTAKE: 98% of US population

TOP 5 RECIPES FOR EPA AND DHA

1. Grilled Wild Salmon with Garlic Scape Pesto = 246% (see page 245)
2. Mussels Three Ways = 200% (see page 239)
3. Whole Trout en Papillote = 140% (see page 249)
4. Garlic Butter Shrimp = 124% (see page 246)
5. Sunflower-Parmesan Crisps = 120% (see page 146)

* There is no established RDA or AI for long-chained PUFAs in the United States. This estimate is based on international recommendations and available data.

Zinc

The basic job of your DNA is to turn food into proteins, and the proteins then serve as the various workers of your body (some proteins facilitate biological reactions, some proteins serve as structural components of cells, etc.). More than 100 of your enzymes use zinc to function—and several of these enzymes aid the translation of DHA into proteins. If DNA is your book of life, zinc-based enzymes act as your reading glasses.

This mineral is also key to your immune function, which is your body's defense system that protects you from infections, cancer, and excess inflammation. Zinc is one of the main reasons you need to eat seafood or meat to eat complete. Plants contain zinc, but they hold on to it quite tightly—so tightly that you don't absorb much. And while grains contain zinc, 80 percent of that zinc is lost when grains are refined, which is another reason you should eat whole grains.

While we routinely check for the levels of many minerals, zinc is not checked. Stress can cause zinc levels to drop, as can illness and heavy exercise. It is nearly impossible to diagnose low levels of zinc. The symptoms are very diverse because it is central to so many functions—your immune system, your ability to burn fats and carbohydrates, even the ability of your cells to divide. Like plants, your body holds on to zinc, mainly storing it in your muscles, with only 0.5 percent of your zinc floating around in your bloodstream.

It's important to note that the human brain, as it develops, is very hungry for zinc, and this mineral is more easily absorbed from human breast milk than from cow's milk. Zinc is so crucial to your health that if you are deficient in it, you also become functionally deficient in vitamin A and folate, two of the other 21 essential nutrients, as zinc is needed for those nutrients to be effective. Taking too much zinc in supplement form can impair immune function and cause GI distress, so there is all the more reason to get the zinc that you need from the food that you eat.

AMOUNT YOU SHOULD EAT PER DAY: Women: 8mg / Men: 11 mg

INSUFFICIENT DIETARY INTAKE: 42% of US population

DEFICIENCY RISK FACTOR: Vegetarian diet, pregnancy and lactation, and heavy alcohol use. Diuretic medication can increase excretion by the kidneys by 60%.

TOP 5 FOOD SOURCES: Oysters (413% in 6 oysters), steak (175% in one 5-oz steak), sesame seeds (34% in ¼ cup), pumpkin seeds (31% in ¼ cup), and ground turkey (23% in 3 oz)

TOP 5 RECIPES

1. Grilled Oyster Tacos = 570% (see page 252)
2. Raw Oysters = 280% (see page 242)
3. Sunday Slow-Cooker Beef Shank = 200% (see page 230)
4. Spicy Shredded Beef Soup = 121% (see page 201)
5. Cast-Iron Steak Dinner with Buttery Cauliflower Mash = 99% (see page 218)

COOKING EFFECT: Soaking beans and legumes increases the availability of zinc, as does letting them sprout.

ABSORPTION: The body absorbs 20–40% of the zinc present in food, but iron supplements impair your absorption of zinc from food.

STORAGE: Zinc is not stored in the body, so your body needs a steady supply.

Vitamin B_{12} (Cobalamin)

B_{12}, the biggest vitamin that you eat, is absorbed and concentrated by animals and seafood. The methyl groups and cobalt that make up this vitamin are woven together by bacteria, which are the only thing that can assemble this vitamin—revealing another way our health is tied to bacteria. There is no vitamin B_{12} in plants, nor can the bacteria in your gut make enough B_{12} to prevent deficiency. Vitamin B_{12}'s size is important as it creates a challenge for your body to absorb and transport. You possess a set of cells lining the stomach whose mission is to ensure the absorption of B_{12}. They excrete a protein called intrinsic factor, which binds to B_{12} and facilitates absorption.

About four times as large as folate or choline, vitamin B_{12} is central to your methylation cycle, a process in which methyl groups, which are single units of carbon, are moved between molecules. If your body had a currency, methyl groups would be the one-dollar bill. Every time your DNA replicates, every time your cells divide, every time there's an electrical impulse in your brain, these methyl groups are transferred in between molecules. As a result, many of your body's functions depend on vitamin B_{12}.

B_{12} is one of two vitamins that predict how fast your brain shrinks as you age. It's a depressing thought, but all brains eventually shrink as you grow older. One key approach to slowing the rate of that shrinkage is to maximize your absorption of vitamin B_{12} by keeping the stomach and gut healthy, and also to eat the most concentrated sources of B_{12}.

Low levels of B_{12} can cause irreversible damage to brain and nerve cells at any age. And an actual B_{12} deficiency causes depression, anemia, and even psychotic symptoms such as extreme paranoia or hearing voices.

You depend on seven B vitamins. They all dissolve in water, which means they need specialized transporters to get into and out of cells through the fatty cell membrane. B_{12} is clearly important, as you store more of it than any of the other B vitamins. You can store only a few weeks' worth of the other B vitamins at a time, but you store several years' worth of B_{12} using a storage mechanism in the liver. While this seems like an excellent insurance policy, B_{12} deficiency is still common in many populations. Vegans and vegetarians are at greatest risk, as meat and animal products like dairy are the only sources of B_{12}. Vegans must take supplements, and vegetarians must rely on dairy and/or supplements.

Deficiency is also common in people over fifty, as some people produce less stomach acid as they age, and this is a crucial element for B_{12} absorption from food. Acid reflux medications also decrease acid production and interfere with the body's ability to absorb B_{12}

Clams and mussels are quite high in B_{12}. Even though these animals cannot make B_{12} in their cells, they are able to save up the B_{12} produced by bacteria and concentrate it in their cells.

AMOUNT YOU SHOULD EAT PER DAY: 2.4mcg for women and men

INSUFFICIENT DIETARY INTAKE: 20% of US population, and 73% of vegans have blood levels that are deficient or insufficient.

TOP FOOD SOURCES: Clams (1,401% in 3 oz), beef liver (1,178% in 3 oz), mussels (833% in 3 oz), sardines (338% in 3 oz), crab (127% in 3 oz), trout (106% in 3 oz), and wild salmon (82% in 3 oz)

TOP 5 RECIPES

1. Mussels Three Ways = 1,125–1,133% (see page 239)
2. Creamy Marsala Wine Pâté = 583% (see page 143)
3. Summer Clam Chowder = 533% (see page 204)
4. Baked Flaxseed Crab Cakes = 417% (see page 254)
5. Grilled Oyster Tacos = 413% (see page 252)

COOKING EFFECT: Extreme heat, boiling for long periods of time, and microwaving can decrease amounts by 30–40%.

ABSORPTION: Damage to the stomach from heavy alcohol use, decreased stomach acidity from acid-blocking medications or aging, pernicious anemia, and autoimmune disease can all interfere with absorption.

STORAGE: The human body stores two to three years' worth of vitamin B_{12} in the liver.

Magnesium

The flow of energy from the sun to your food to you begins with the mineral magnesium. This element is at the center of photosynthesis—the process by which plants turn sunlight into sugar—and is therefore foundational to life on the planet and our entire food supply.

In terms of your body, magnesium is required for the proper function of nerve cells and brain cells. It also helps relax the smooth muscle that lines your blood vessels, thereby decreasing blood pressure.

Magnesium is one of the few nutrients that directly stimulate brain growth. Thus eating for brain health requires adding more magnesium-rich foods to your diet, such as beans, nuts, and leafy greens. Magnesium also helps control blood sugar, and diets with higher levels of magnesium are associated with lower risk of diabetes.

Inside your cells, magnesium acts as a cofactor, which means that critical molecular pathways depend on this mineral—pathways that build healthy cells, efficiently deal with waste, and slow your aging. A biochemical pathway

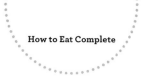

is just like a recipe: basic ingredients are combined and transformed into something more complex. Magnesium is a key ingredient in your body's chemistry, affecting everything from the production of DNA to the electricity in your brain cells.

Magnesium was the very first mental health intervention tested in a scientific trial. In 1922, a group of patients with "agitated depression" were given an IV infusion of magnesium. A few hours later, all the people in the study were calm and many were actually asleep. Magnesium is a calming balm, the key to helping you relax.

AMOUNT YOU SHOULD EAT PER DAY: Women: 320mg / Men: 420mg

INSUFFICIENT DIETARY INTAKE: 68% of US population

DEFICIENCY RISK FACTORS: Gastrointestinal diseases, type 2 diabetes, and alcohol dependence

TOP 5 FOOD SOURCES: Almonds (25% in 1 oz), spinach (24% in ½ cup), cashews (23% in 1 oz), black beans (19% in ½ cup), and soybeans (16% in ½ cup)

TOP 5 RECIPES

1. Kiwi Green Smoothie = 80% (see page 113)
2. Minty Blueberry Shake = 75% (see page 115)
3. Crispy Shrimp with Greens and Beans = 55% (see page 257)
4. Chocolate Hot Amaranth Breakfast Cereal = 49% (see page 129)
5. Mussels with Garlicky Kale Ribbons = 48% (see page 239)

COOKING EFFECT: Boiling foods that contain magnesium can cause 20–30% loss of the magnesium level.

ABSORPTION: Net absorption is about 50%, but a high-fiber diet actually decreases absorption.

STORAGE: An adult body contains approximately 25g of magnesium.

Vitamin B₉ (Folate)

The word *folate* comes from *folium*, the Latin word for "foliage," which gives you an easy reminder of one place to find this vitamin: in leafy greens. Folate is the natural form of folic acid and serves as another workhorse for your body. It is critical for the regulation of your DNA and the production of key building blocks in your brain. Folate is needed to make myelin (the insulation around your neurons) and major neurotransmitters such as serotonin, dopamine, and norepinephrine. These important chemicals regulate your mood, your sense of pleasure, and the clarity of your thinking.

Low levels of folate cause low mood and low energy and can speed the aging of your brain, thereby putting you at risk for cognitive decline. Low intake of folate during pregnancy can disrupt the formation of the brain and spinal cord of a fetus. Because dietary intake of folate went down as we started eating more processed food, folic acid was added to flour as a public health intervention.

Folate is required for a key step in the formation of SAMe, a substance in the brain that is a key to making just about everything: DNA, serotonin, myelin, and more. SAMe has been used with some success to treat clinical depression. In addition, folate processes an amino acid called homocysteine in your body. When homocysteine in your blood is high, it is a general marker of inflammation in your body, a sign that the gears of your cells aren't turning smoothly—and that you don't have enough folate to process the homocystiene. High homosystiene is a serious risk factor for depression, dementia, and heart disease. Folate helps lubricate those gears, thereby preventing high levels.

AMOUNT YOU SHOULD EAT PER DAY: 400mcg for women and men

INSUFFICIENT DIETARY INTAKE: 75% of US population

TOP FOOD SOURCES: Chicken liver (120% in 3 oz), lentils (90% in 1 cup), chickpeas (71% in 1 cup), black-eyed peas (54% in 1 cup), Brussels sprouts (40% in 1 cup), asparagus (22% in 4 spears), and cooked spinach (15% in 1 cup)

TOP 5 RECIPES

    1. Citrus Scallops = 136% (see page 148)
    2. Creamy Marsala Wine Pâté = 136% (see page 143)
    3. Pancetta Brussels Sprouts = 82% (see page 151)
    4. Artichoke-Leek Carpaccio = 68% (see page 141)
    5. Mussels with Garlicky Kale Ribbons = 56% (see page 239)

COOKING EFFECT: Folate is heat and light sensitive, which is one reason to get your greens fresh and eat them raw. When you cook greens, make it a quick sauté, as extended cooking can reduce the amount of folate by 50–75%. And never boil your greens; this destroys folate and other health-promoting compounds such as heat-sensitive phytonutrients. Freezing, on the other hand, does not affect folate content, so frozen foods are a great source when fresh produce is out of season.

ABSORPTION: Crohn's disease and alcoholism may decrease absorption.

STORAGE: The human body contains 10–30mg of folate, with about half of that stored in the liver.

Good Bugs: Prebiotics and Probiotics

Your overall health depends on your gut health for the absorption of the nutrients you need. But there is more to the story. Today, we recognize another role of your gut as home to a bacteria population known to influence your immune and nervous systems. Based on recent research, the bacteria that populate your gut are implicated in your mood, how clearly you think, and how anxious you are. Prebiotics are the fiber in food that is consumed by the bacteria in your gut, and probiotics are foods that contain live bacteria.

You have about ten times more bacterial cells in your body than human cells. While your human cells have only 23,000 genes, the bacteria in your gut are estimated to have over two million genes. This collection of genetic material is called the microbiome. For centuries in medicine we have tried to kill bacteria because they cause infection. But today, we know there is a more complex biological picture to paint. The bacteria, yeasts, and fungi that live in and on your body dictate much about your health. With so much to learn,

The National Institutes of Health launched the Human Microbiome Project in 2008. To date the project has identified more than 10,000 species of bacteria that populate the human gut, but most people have 500 to 1,000 species. The most common species in your gut is *Faecalibacterium prausnitzii*, which is about 5 percent of the bacterial population. About 60 percent of the mass of your stool is actually bacteria.

The bacteria of interest are not those that cause disease, such as *E. coli*, but those referred to as commensals. These bacteria live in harmony with us. After you absorb all the nutrients you can in your small intestine, the indigestible fibers enter the colon. This is where more energy is extracted by the bacteria, which can ferment and digest these fibers. It is estimated that about 15 percent of your total energy is derived from this salvaging of calories by the bacteria in your colon.

And your gut does more than digest food. It is the biggest organ in your immune system, and the species of bacteria in your microbiome have a great influence on that immune system as a result. This has large implications for autoimmune illnesses, which are on the rise, as well as neuropsychiatric brain illnesses such as depression and autism. Some gut microbes are known to cause cancer, others help train the immune system, and "healthy" bugs keep the growth of bacteria that cause illness in check. A healthy microbiome protects the lining of the gut and promotes a healthy intestinal barrier. Having certain bacteria in your gut can either protect against or promote weight gain and obesity. And the brain and the gut speak a common language: the neurotransmitters serotonin, dopamine, and GABA are all produced by bacteria in the gut.

The complexity of gut bacteria's influence on our health can be a bit overwhelming. Thankfully, a summary of the science results in two simple steps for you as an eater: seed them and feed them. This means that you seed the gut, first at birth and by breast-feeding, and then later in life by ingesting more live bacterial cultures in fermented foods like yogurt, kefir, and pickled vegetables such as sauerkraut. These foods all contain various species of bacteria associated with health benefits, namely species of *Lactobacillus* or *Bifidobacterium*. Foods that contain live bacteria cultures are "probiotics." While this helps get the right bacteria into your gut, the only way to really shift your microbiome towards health is eating more fiber—which means more plants. Bacteria break down fiber into short-chained fatty acids, which are nourishment for the human cells that line your intestines. They can also create some vitamins, such as vitamin K_2 and several B vitamins. People who eat a more traditional plant-based diet have higher counts of these health-promoting bacteria and a lower incidence of bacteria that cause disease.

Broadly, there are two categories of fiber: soluble fiber that dissolves in water, and insoluble fiber that does not and is largely inert. Insoluble fibers absorb water and add bulk to stool. They also help you feel full longer after a meal. Both kinds can be "prebiotics," meaning they are digested and fermented by bacteria. Certain kinds of fiber are preferred by certain bacteria. Eating more of the prebiotic fiber increases the population of protective, health-promoting good bugs like *Bacteriodes*, while refined grains and sugars facilitate the growth of disease-causing bacteria like *E. coli* and *C. difficile*. The microbiome thus changes slightly after each meal, and studies of dietary change have shown significant shifts in the kinds of bacteria and how they function in a few weeks.

AMOUNT YOU SHOULD EAT PER DAY: Women: 25g / Men: 38g of fiber. There is no established recommended intake for probiotics.

INSUFFICIENT DIETARY INTAKE: 97% of US population

TOP 5 FOOD SOURCES (FIBER): Navy beans (76% in 1 cup), lentils (63% in 1 cup), tempeh (48% in 1 cup), raspberries (32% in 1 cup), and collard greens (30% in 1 cup)

TOP RECIPES (FIBER)

1. Artichoke-Leek Carpaccio = 92% (see page 141)
2. Kiwi Green Smoothie = 80% (see page 113)
3. Black Bean Salad = 78% (see page 188)
4. Rainbow Burgers = 68% (see page 161)
5. Cacao Nib–Pepita Granola = 48% (see page 134)
6. Scallop-Shrimp Ceviche with Pickled Ginger and Radishes = 48% (see page 250)

TOP 5 RECIPES (PROBIOTICS)
1. Homemade Kefir with Apples (see page 127)
2. Gingered Pumpkin Smoothie (see page 118)
3. Balsamic Strawberry Parfait (see page 119)
4. Minty Blueberry Shake (see page 115)
5. Kiwi Green Smoothie (see page 113)

COOKING EFFECT: Cooking kills most live cultures.

ABSORPTION: Fiber and probiotic bacteria are not absorbed by the body.

STORAGE: Your body does not store fiber. Your gut contains trillions of bacteria.

Complete Proteins

Protein is essential to your diet because it provides the building blocks for the thousands of parts in your body: enzymes, cell receptors, and cell scaffolding are all made of amino acids. When you eat proteins, your body breaks them down into amino acids, absorbs them, and then uses them to build your own proteins. If you think of your DNA as a recipe book, your genes give you the instructions to cook up a vast array of proteins, and amino acids are their basic ingredient.

The long chains of amino acids are broken down during digestion by the acids in your stomach as a well as enzymes in your saliva. Your pancreas secretes enzymes that further break proteins down into amino acids, which are absorbed by specific transporters in the small intestine. The proteins that make up your body are constantly being replaced as you resynthesize about 250 grams of protein every day. It makes sense then that protein needs vary by weight. You need 0.8 gram of protein per kilogram of body weight per day.

If your diet is missing an amino acid or two, your body has the ability to convert some amino acids into others. But the essential amino acids are the ones you don't have the ability to make, meaning you must consume them as part of your diet instead. Of the twenty amino acids, nine are essential: histidine, isoleucine, leucine, lysine, methionine, phenylalanine, threonine, tryptophan, and valine. For example, tryptophan is the building block of the neurotransmitter serotonin, so as the levels of tryptophan in the brain drop, the rate of serotonin production drops. This generally leads to a lower mood, memory impairment, and often more aggression. Countries in which people eat more tryptophan have lower rates of suicide.

All meats, seafood, dairy, and eggs come with complete protein, meaning they come with all nine essential amino acids. Plants, especially beans, other legumes, and nuts, can be good sources of protein, and if eaten in the right combinations can provide all nine essential amino acids.

Today, many people eat much more protein than needed, almost double what's needed for the average American man. So if people eat too much protein, why focus on this nutrient? First off, many eaters need to expand their use of plant-based proteins in place of excess meat and also upgrade the quality of the meat they eat. Red meat makes up 58 percent of the meat consumption in the United States and processed meats account for another 22 percent. There are some health risks associated with this pattern, along with environmental costs. Second, focusing on protein quality guides us to proteins that are more digestible and contain more of the nine essential amino acids. The Protein Digestibility Corrected Amino Acid Score (PDCAAS) is a way of ranking proteins based on the essential amino acids and how well they are digested. Milk and dairy proteins, eggs, soy protein, and meat top the list. Finally, there are two amino acids of particular importance to brain health: tryptophan and tyrosine. It is not as simple as "eat more tryptophan and be happier," but you should know that the amino acid tryptophan is the most rare amino acid in food. That's why I also included the top recipes for this amino acid. Taking L-tryptophan as a supplement led to a number of deaths from a rare condition called Eosinophilia-Myalgia Syndrome (EMS) in 1989. This was caused by a contaminant, and led to the supplement being banned in the United States. While it's back on the market now, there have been subsequent cases of EMS, and food remains the best way to increase tryptophan intake.

AMOUNT YOU SHOULD EAT PER DAY: Women: 46g / Men: 56g

INSUFFICIENT DIETARY INTAKE: 8% of adolescent girls and older women in the US

TOP FOOD SOURCES: Animal sources (per 3 oz cooked): turkey (54%), chicken (43%), salmon (37%), beef (77%), liver (37%); plant sources (per 1 cup cooked): soybeans (67%), tofu (48%), lentils (39%), white beans (37%), kidney beans (37%)

TOP 5 RECIPES

Animal Sources
1. Sunday Slow-Cooker Beef Shank = 124% (see page 230)
2. Whole Roasted Chicken with Anchovies and Olives = 113% (see page 210)
3. Cast-Iron Steak Dinner with Buttery Cauliflower Mash = 100% (see page 218)
4. Crispy Shrimp with Greens and Beans = 83% (see page 257)
5. Pan-Roasted Duck and Potatoes with Cherry Sauce = 80% (see page 232)

Plant Sources
1. Balsamic Strawberry Parfait = 56% (see page 119)
2. Minty Blueberry Shake = 50% (see page 115)
3. Kiwi Green Smoothie = 43% (see page 113)
4. Lazy Green Mac and Cheese = 41% (see page 162)
5. Black Rice with Grilled Radicchio = 41% (see page 158)

Tryptophan
1. Whole Roasted Chicken with Anchovies and Olives = 590mg (see page 210)
2. Sunday Slow-Cooker Beef Shank = 574mg (see page 230)
3. Pan-Roasted Duck and Potatoes with Cherry Sauce = 504mg (see page 232)
4. Pumpkin Seed–Crusted Lamb Chops = 405mg (see page 226)
5. Spicy Shredded Beef Soup = 388mg (see page 201)

COOKING EFFECT: Heat increases the digestibility of protein.

ABSORPTION: Absorption depends on stomach acid and digestive enzymes.

STORAGE: Proteins make up 20% of your body mass, especially muscle.

7 FOR PROTECTION

Vitamin E

Vitamin E is a firefighter. Every second, thousands of "fires" erupt on the surface of your cells, and the dedicated job of vitamin E is to put those fires out. Your brain is particularly vulnerable to fires because it contains high concentrations of omega-3 fats, and these fats are very easy to oxidize. (This is why fish, with its high omega-3 content, spoils faster than other meats.) Oxidation is the process of adding electrons, usually from oxygen, to any molecule. Just as the oxidation of a wildfire spreads the fire, so can oxidation in a cell. For example "free radicals" are unstable molecules with a single unpaired electron that are produced when your cell's powerhouses turn food fuel into cell fuel. Free radicals promote oxidation, which is why we look to antioxidants to counter them. As vitamin E is a fat-soluble antioxidant, it is uniquely suited to protect the outer layer of fat that surrounds each of your cells. By dissolving in the fat that makes up the cell membrane, it protects cells from oxidative damage in a way that other antioxidants can't.

Given the brain's inherent vulnerability, it is worrisome that more people are missing this vitamin than any other: 96 percent of eaters don't meet the daily requirement of vitamin E. The fats that make up your cell membranes influence everything from the sharpness of your brain to the glow of your skin, and your body depends on having vitamin E to protect those fats. Vitamin E also protects the brain by triggering the relaxation of blood vessels and making blood less "sticky," which helps decrease inflammation. Low vitamin E greatly increases the risk of depression and dementia.

In whole foods there are actually eight forms of vitamin E, grouped into the tocopherols and the tocotrienols. Fortified foods and supplements use only one form—alpha-tocopherol—which is the most common in your body. But it should be noted that the alpha-tocopherol found in whole foods has twice the biological potency, literally twice the power, of the form found in supplements—yet another reason to get your nutrients from natural sources whenever possible. Plus, natural foods offer all eight forms of the vitamin E family.

High amounts of vitamin E are found in few food sources. Given its protective function, researchers have tested vitamin E supplements for a variety of health conditions. Unfortunately, studies of vitamin E supplementation "have been a disaster," in the words of one of my colleagues. While more natural vitamin E in your diet is strongly correlated with lower risk of heart disease, dementia, and cancer, studies of vitamin E supplements show little effect and actually suggest some harm.

AMOUNT YOU SHOULD EAT PER DAY: 15mg for women and men

INSUFFICIENT DIETARY INTAKE: 96% of US population

TOP 5 FOOD SOURCES: Sunflower seeds (82% in ¼ cup), almonds (40% in ¼ cup), spinach (25% in 1 cup), avocado (21% in 1 cup), and olive oil (13% in 1 tbsp)

TOP 5 RECIPES
1. Clove-Spiked Cocktail Nut Mix = 40% (see page 144)
2. Flourless Chocolate-Almond Cake = 30% (see page 279)
3. Buttermilk Strawberry Smoothie = 30% (see page 117)
4. Gingered Pumpkin Smoothie = 20% (see page 118)
5. Mixed Nut–Cardamon Baklava Bites = 20% (see page 278)

COOKING EFFECT: Heating and long-term storage can decrease vitamin E.

ABSORPTION: Increased by fats.

STORAGE: Your body does not store vitamin E. Tissue concentrations are dependent on intake.

Vitamin K

Vitamin K is not a vitamin many people consider when making food choices. Named for its role in the coagulation of blood (it was discovered in Germany, the "k" coming from *Koagulierung*), this is a family of five known forms of the vitamin (to date). Its role, regulating blood coagulation and clotting, helps ensure your brain receives oxygen, a delicate task as small leaks must be instantly plugged without compromising blood flow. Vitamin K is key to bone formation and is also a cofactor for the enzymes that help determine if your arteries calcify, a step in the development of heart disease.

While the role of vitamin K in the brain is just emerging, we know the brain possesses high concentrations of a particular version of vitamin K_2, called MK–4. It serves an integral role in the construction of the very specialized fats that insulate your brain cells and allow for the ultrarapid communication between cells. A diet with higher intake of K_2 is correlated with a decreased risk of heart disease, premature death, and severe calcification of the arteries. A recent large epidemiological study that followed 7,216 people for four years found that people who increased their vitamin K intake had a reduction in the risk of cancer by 59 percent and the risk of heart disease by 48 percent, compared with participants who did not increase their vitamin K intake.

Choosing foods high in vitamin K means basing your diet on the most foundational element of the food supply, the leaf. Greens such as kale, Swiss chard, and spinach are all very high in vitamin K_1, phylloquinone. Vitamin K_2 (menoquinone) is found in fermented foods, as these forms are made by bacteria. K_2 is stored in the liver, making liver meat another good source. The bacteria in your microbiome also produce some vitamin K_2 for you.

AMOUNT YOU SHOULD EAT PER DAY: Women: 90mcg / Men: 120 mcg

INSUFFICIENT DIETARY INTAKE: 75% of US population*

TOP 5 FOOD SOURCES: Kale (1,180% in 1 cup), spinach (987% in 1 cup), mustard greens (922% in 1 cup), collard greens (858% in 1 cup), and beet greens (774% in 1 cup)

TOP 5 RECIPES
1. Citrus Scallops = 1,317% (see page 148)
2. Marinated Kale Salad = 699% (see page 177)
3. Hearty Winter Kale Salad = 649% (see page 173)
4. Mussels with Garlicky Kale Ribbons = 631% (see page 239)
5. Baked Eggs in Crispy Kale Cups = 610% (see page 126)

COOKING EFFECT: Vitamin K is stable for most types of processing. Cooking generally increases concentrations, but decreases water content.

ABSORPTION: Absorption of vitamin K is greatly increased by adding fats such as olive oil, and impaired by GI disorders such as ulcerative colitis or after bariatric surgery.

STORAGE: Your body has a very limited capacity to store vitamin K and levels begin to decline in about 10 days without intake.

* Adequate Intake cannot technically be used to calculate dietary insufficiency. This is based on a USDA statement that only one in four Americans meets the AI.

Vitamin A and Carotenoids

Vitamin A and its carotenoid precursors teach us about our connection to plants. Carotenoids absorb light. Much as plants use light to drive their metabolism by making sugar from sunlight, we use carotenoids to harness light and create our sense of vision. We are able to make vitamin A from a number of pigments in plants, mainly the abundant orange and yellow ones such as beta-carotene. Fully formed vitamin A, known as retinol, is found only in meat, eggs, and dairy.

As one of the four vitamins that dissolve and work in fat, vitamin A plays a critical role in the brain and body. Like many of the essential vitamins, vitamin A regulates cell growth and division and also helps maintain everything from your immune system to the health of your skin. Carotenoids are a large family of 600 plant pigments, and a few, such as beta-carotene, are converted to the active form of vitamin A in your body called retinol. Vitamin A receptors are found throughout the brain but particularly near genes that influence mood and memory. Vitamin A also plays a role in your ability to produce DHA, the longest omega-3 fat and a key building block of the brain.

The other carotenoids play a role in our health, too. Several, such as lycopene, are known to travel to the brain, where they serve as antioxidants and appear to protect the brain by decreasing inflammation. They seem to protect very specialized, energy-demanding cells like the nerve cells that make up your eyes and brain. Lutein and zeaxanthin protect your vision and prevent macular degeneration, the top cause of blindness later in life.

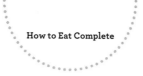

Higher levels of carotenoids are correlated with a lower risk of dementia. While food forms of carotenoids are also correlated with lower cancer risk, it is important to note that beta-carotene supplements appear to be harmful, especially in smokers.

Vitamin A stores are highly variable, but by eating a diet high in carotenoids as well as the top dietary sources of retinol, you can ensure healthy levels. Excess retinol can be toxic, though this has been reported only from supplemented vitamin A, never from food sources. Retinol is rapidly absorbed and is cleared from the body slowly, thereby making it possible to obtain toxically high levels via supplements. On the other end of the spectrum, a vitamin A deficiency can cause night blindness, though this is rare in the developed world.

AMOUNT YOU SHOULD EAT PER DAY: Women: 700mcg / Men: 900mcg

RATE OF INSUFFICIENT INTAKE: 40% of US men, 32% of US women

TOP 5 FOOD SOURCES: Sweet potato (438% in 1 medium potato), carrots (428% in 1 cup), pumpkin (245% in 1 cup), chicken liver (186% in 3 oz), and mustard greens (118% in 1 cup)

TOP 5 RECIPES

1. Creamy Marsala Wine Pâté = 444% (see page 143)
2. Paprika Shrimp with Peppadew Peppers = 212% (see page 251)
3. Summer Clam Chowder = 195% (see page 204)
4. Gingered Pumpkin Smoothie = 179% (see page 118)
5. Rainbow Burgers = 168% (see page 161)

COOKING EFFECT: Vitamin A as retinol is relatively stable in animal foods; for some foods, such as tomatoes, carotenoids are more easily absorbed after processing: e.g., tomato paste contains more than the whole tomato form.

ABSORPTION: Increased with the addition of fats; e.g., olive oil, eggs, and nuts.

STORAGE: Your body's stores of vitamin A in your liver depend on your intake. You use 0.5% of your stores daily.

Phytonutrients: The Polyphenols

Phytonutrients are molecules from plants (*phyto* = plant). There are thousands of these nutrients in nature and their impact on our health is an active area of research. Plants use these molecules to combat the damage of UVB radiation (which is why eating more lycopene increases the SPF of your skin) and to help themselves fight off invaders. This means many of these phytonutrients have the ability to fight bacteria, viruses, and fungi.

The largest family of phytonutrients is called polyphenols, which refers to their chemical structure and shape, and more than 8,000 of these have been identified in nature. In general, polyphenols are large molecules. There are many different types of polyphenols—for example, the flavonoids, phenolic acids, anthocyanins, and lignans. These vary in their absorption, human biological activity, and the amount of evidence we have on how they work. The anthocyanins are pigment molecules that impart a red, blue, or purple color to plants. As a general rule, the more darkly colored the fruit, the more of anthocyanins it contains. Also part of the broad category of phytonutrients are the carotenoids, which (as mentioned above) are best known for their role as vitamin A precursors, though they also have antioxidant, protective, and cell regulation functions.

Consumption of polyphenols is associated with a decreased risk of the chronic illnesses that plague modern societies, such as heart disease, diabetes, and cancer. Yet the biggest promise of these molecules may be their effect on brain growth. A number of polyphenols from cacao, blueberries, green tea, turmeric, and onions can promote the expression of brain growth factor BDNF and have strong antioxidant effects in the brain. Even though the science of how these molecules affect our brain health is still emerging, it is compelling enough to justify boosting your intake of a variety of plants.

Because these molecules are used by the plant for protection, you find the highest concentrations in the skin and outer layers. This is one reason that eating whole fruits and vegetables is better than drinking juice. For example, eating an orange gives you five times the flavonoid polyphenols compared with a glass of orange juice.

The amounts of different polyphenols vary depending on the plant, the

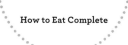

growth environment, and the level of ripeness. One reason I recommend that people "eat the rainbow" is that the many colors represent eating a diverse set of polyphenols and carotenoids. Generally, organic foods have higher levels of polyphenols, as these plants are more "stressed" by invaders and so produce more defenses.

Absorption of many polyphenols depends on bacteria in the gut, as the complex molecules are modified by bacteria. Some research also suggests that certain polyphenols stay in our bodies by getting absorbed by the gut, metabolized by the liver, and then excreted into the gut again in bile and reabsorbed.

AMOUNT YOU SHOULD EAT PER DAY: No established recommendation

RATE OF INSUFFICIENT INTAKE: 80% of US population does not meet recommendation of 5 or more servings of fruits and vegetables per day. Fruit and vegetable consumption declined by 7% from 2004 to 2009.

TOP FOOD SOURCES: Polyphenol content and absorption vary widely. In general, smaller, more darkly colored fruits, vegetables, and seeds have the highest contents.

TOP 5 RECIPES

1. Rainbow Burgers (see page 161)
2. Hearty Winter Kale Salad with Purple Potatoes and Hemp Seeds (see page 173)
3. Black Rice with Radiccio, Beets, and Goat Cheese (see page 158)
4. Sourdough Bueberry Pancakes with Kiwi–Red Currant Sauce (see page 130)
5. Quinoa-Mushroom Frittata with Fresh Herbs (see page 120)

COOKING EFFECT: Peeling vegetables greatly reduces polyphenol content. Many polyphenols are heat sensitive. Boiling causes 80% loss. Steaming results in minimal loss.

ABSORPTION: Varies greatly for different polyphenols.

STORAGE: You have no system to store phytonutrients. Those that dissolve in fat are incorporated into cell membranes.

Monounsaturated Fats (MUFAs)

These fats are not as flexible or prone to oxidation as polyunsaturated fats, but they are more fluid than saturated fats. One thing I like about these fats is the lack of controversy: MUFAs are considered quite healthy. These fats are one of the factors that define the Mediterranean diet.

OLEIC ACID. This is the most abundant fat in many things we eat: olive oil, beef, fish, almonds, and even lard. It is strongly linked to a decreased risk of heart disease, diabetes, and depression. Eating more oleic acid improves insulin sensitivity, meaning your body is more efficient at metabolizing sugars. The only clinical trial in humans that followed levels of Brain Derived Neurotrophic Factor (BDNF), the growth factor that enhances brain health, found that participants whose diets were augmented with nuts were 78 percent less likely to have severely low levels of BDNF. Oleic acid is also used by the body to create oleoylethanolamide, which enhances memory, induces fat burning, promotes weight loss, and reduces appetite.

NERVONIC ACID. This fat is not a large part of your diet, but it is linked to a number of mental health conditions. It is a primary component of myelin, the insulation of your brain cells that dramatically increases the speed of neuron signal transmission and is essential to brain function. Lower levels of this fat are found in children with ADHD and in patients with treatment-resistant clinical depression. Nervonic acid is linked to a decreased risk of obesity and of heart disease. You'll find this fat in salmon, mustard, human breast milk, flaxseed oil, and hemp seeds.

VACCENIC ACID. This fat is made in the stomach of ruminants such as cattle and sheep and is found in higher concentrations in grass-fed meat and dairy products. Your body converts it to rumenic acid, a CLA fat that decreases body fat, increases muscle mass, and prevents metabolic syndrome. Vaccenic acid is a natural trans fat, but unlike those in processed foods, this natural trans fat has documented health-promoting and anticancer effects.

AMOUNT YOU SHOULD EAT PER DAY: This should be the primary fat in your diet, between 300 and 500 calories per day.

INSUFFICIENT DIETARY INTAKE: 80% of US population

TOP 5 FOOD SOURCES: Olive oil, almonds, avocados, nut butters, cashews

TOP 5 RECIPES

1. Grilled Summer Bounty = 24g (see page 178)
2. Rocket Pie = 16g (see page 237)
3. Beet Greens with Homemade Citrus Wild Salmon Gravlax = 15g (see page 183)
4. Berry-Spinach Salad = 15g (see page 181)
5. Grilled Chicken with Asparagus-Almond-Tarragon Pesto = 14g (see page 214)

COOKING EFFECT: Depending on quality, olive oil has a smoke point from 370 to 450 degrees Fahrenheit. High heat damages the polyphenols and degrades the fat.

ABSORPTION: MUFAs are readily absorbed.

STORAGE: The human body is made of MUFAs, which are an important fat in every cell of your body.

Vitamin D

Vitamin D deficiency is now recognized as a pandemic.
—Michael F. Holick, MD, PhD, Boston University School of Medicine

Vitamin D deficiency is widespread, with profound negative health consequences ranging from brittle bones to a fragile brain. Vitamin D is one of the four fat-soluble vitamins, and one of the original complex molecules on the planet: phytoplankton in the ocean make it when exposed to sunlight, as do mushrooms. Vitamin D is not essential, as you make it when your skin uses UVB rays of sunlight to create vitamin D from cholesterol. But this is still the most common vitamin deficiency I see in my practice. Sunscreen blocks 99 percent of vitamin D production in the skin, and as we spend more time inside, our sun exposure is at an all-time low. Our needs are also higher, as obesity contributes to deficiency by increasing need.

Vitamin D is actually a hormone. It influences cells all over your body because being fat soluble means it can glide through the fatty cell membranes and interact with your DNA. Consider for a moment that when you eat vitamin D, it travels from the end of your fork all the way to the center of your cells, where it "talks" to your DNA.

This vitamin is critical for helping you use calcium to build your bones and keep them strong. It's of concern that many women taking a calcium supplement are vitamin D deficient and so cannot effectively absorb or use calcium. Vitamin D also has a role regulating the immune system, and may play a role in preventing high blood pressure and certain cancers.

Vitamin D is deeply involved in brain health. Low levels and deficiencies accelerate brain aging and are correlated with a worsening of diseases that affect the brain, such as depression and multiple sclerosis.

The most common form of vitamin D in supplements and fortified food is ergocalciferol, known as D_2. This is the form also found in plants and is not as biologically potent as cholecalciferol, vitamin D_3, found in animals and in some supplements. While considered equivalent, D_3 is substantially more potent and biologically active than D_2 and about five times more powerful in raising blood levels. In clinical trials, only vitamin D_3 has been shown to prevent fractures.

AMOUNT YOU SHOULD EAT PER DAY: 15mcg for women and men

INSUFFICIENT DIETARY INTAKE: 85–90% of US adolescents, 80% of US adults. (41.6% of Americans are frankly deficient, while 82% of African-Americans and 69% of US Hispanics are deficient.)

TOP 5 FOOD SOURCES: Wild salmon (112% in 3 oz), trout (108% in 3 oz), sardines (26% in 3 oz), tuna (39% in 4 oz), and pork ribs (15% in 3 oz)

TOP 5 RECIPES

1. Grilled Wild Salmon with Garlic Scape Pesto = 200% (see page 245)
2. Sunflower-Parmesan Crisps = 67% (see page 146)
3. Cashew-Chocolate Smoothie = 41% (see page 116)
4. Deviled Green Eggs with Roasted Red Pepper = 40% (see page 153)
5. Quinoa-Mushroom Frittata with Fresh Herbs = 32% (see page 120)

COOKING EFFECT: High-heat cooking may reduce the nutrient amount.

ABSORPTION: Deficiency is more frequent in northern latitudes.

STORAGE: Stores depend on sun exposure and dietary intake.

Selenium

The most powerful antioxidants in your body are not the ones that you eat, but the ones that you make. Coded in your DNA is glutathione, the top antioxidant in your brain, and its production relies on selenium. There are a number of specialized proteins in the body called selenoproteins that require selenium. These proteins make this mineral key to your metabolism, as it too is needed for proper functioning of the thyroid. Your thyroid gland can't use iodine without the assistance of selenoproteins. It is easy to ensure you have both selenium and iodine, as the top food for these nutrients is seafood.

Selenium is needed for reproduction and DNA synthesis, as well as offering protection from oxidative damage. Excess selenium can be toxic, though the only food of concern is Brazil nuts. Signs of high selenium include brittle nails, hair loss, garlicky breath odor, irritability, and fatigue.

AMOUNT YOU SHOULD EAT PER DAY: 55mcg for women and men

INSUFFICIENT DIETARY INTAKE: 15% of US population

TOP 5 FOOD SOURCES: Brazil nuts (1,158% in ¼ cup), lobster (172% in 1 lb lobster), tuna (167% in 3 oz), shrimp (102% in 4 oz), and halibut (85% in 3 oz)

TOP 5 RECIPES

1. Mussels Three Ways = 185–187% (see page 239)
2. Clove-Spiked Cocktail Nut Mix = 169% (see page 144)
3. Chipotle Pork Loin with Blueberry-Kiwi Salsa = 102% (see page 221)
4. Garlic Butter Shrimp = 100% (see page 246)
5. Spicy Shredded Beef Soup = 93% (see page 201)

COOKING EFFECT: For selenium found in meat, processing does not affect the amount by much; however, refining whole wheat reduces selenium content by 45%.

ABSORPTION: Highly absorbable.

STORAGE: No storage. Body stores are in selenoproteins.

7 FOR IGNITION

Iron

Iron is arguably the element most critical to brain function, as it is responsible for binding and transporting oxygen to every cell in your brain and body so that your cells can create energy. Iron is a central part of both hemoglobin, the protein in your blood that transports oxygen; and myoglobin, the iron-based protein in your muscles that stores oxygen for when you need a burst of energy.

Along with being important for transporting oxygen, iron is a key ingredient in the production of the molecules most responsible for mood, focus, and pleasure—namely, dopamine and serotonin. Iron is also needed to make myelin, the fatty layer covering your brain cells that is responsible for ultrafast signal conduction. Brains with less iron have less myelin. And iron is at the center of true detox, as the complex detoxification pathways in your liver rely on this mineral.

Since iron has such an important role to play, you can imagine the sad state a body would be in with a low supply of iron. Low iron can cause incapacitating low energy, a foggy brain, and sadness. Performance of all types—physical, mental, and emotional—can tank when iron levels dip. Women are at risk of low iron due to iron loss during menses, and 10 to 15 percent of women are iron deficient during pregnancy, when the demand for iron increases by 50 percent. Demand also skyrockets during times of growth spurts in early childhood and adolescence. Deficiency during early brain development from conception to the age of three can lead to irreversible problems, including difficulty focusing and decreased intelligence. Kids with low iron tend to be more anxious and hesitant as well.

Periods of high iron demand are of particular concern for vegetarians, as the iron found in plants is 30 to 40 percent less absorbable than the heme iron found in meat and seafood. Plants hold on to their iron very tightly.

But absorption of iron from plants is increased when you eat heme iron in animals, a synergy that suggests humans are likely meant to be omnivores. One benefit of adding acids such as lemon juice when you are cooking plants is an increase in the absorption of iron. Still, even with heme iron, only about 25 percent of the iron you eat is absorbed.

Health officials estimate that two billion people on the planet are iron deficient, and that if this was reversed, the IQ on Earth would increase by 13 points. Are you struggling to perform at work? Sapped of energy? Missing your laser-sharp focus? Time to top off your stores of iron.

Iron Tips

- Eat a mix of animal and plant sources of iron.
- Bivalves (clams, mussels, and oysters) are the top nutritional source of iron, but dark chocolate contains a good dose as well.
- Taking medications that decrease stomach acidity also decreases iron absorption.
- You can increase iron absorption from plants 2 to 6 times by adding acid such as lemon juice.
- The following block iron absorption: phytates in legumes and grains, polyphenol antioxidants and tannins (such as tea and wine), calcium supplements, and soybean vegetable protein.
- The following increase iron need: exercise, infection, pregnancy, periods of growth, and heavy menses.

AMOUNT YOU SHOULD EAT PER DAY: Women: 18mg (during pregnancy: 27 mg) / Men: 8 mg

INSUFFICIENT DIETARY INTAKE: 20% of women ages 31 to 50 in the US.

TOP 5 FOOD SOURCES: Pumpkin seeds (47% in ¼ cup), oysters (44% in 3 oz), dark chocolate (39% in 3 oz), sesame seeds (29% in ¼ cup), and spinach (17% in ½ cup)

TOP 5 RECIPES

1. Pumpkin Seed–Crusted Lamb Chops = 69% (see page 226)
2. Citrus Scallops = 61% (see page 148)
3. Mussels with Garlicky Kale Ribbons = 61% (see page 239)

> 4. Pan-Roasted Duck with Cherry Sauce = 58% (see page 232)
> 5. Mussels with Heirloom Tomatoes = 57% (see page 239)
>
> COOKING EFFECT: Boiling vegetables for long periods of time with a large amount of water can cause up to a 90% iron loss.
>
> ABSORPTION: Heme iron about 25% absorbed, nonheme iron about 17%.
>
> STORAGE: The human body contains on average about 3.5g of iron.

Vitamin B₁ (Thiamine)

Your brain is a furnace with high energy demands, and getting that energy depends on this B vitamin. The brain mainly runs on glucose (blood sugar), and turning glucose into energy requires thiamine.

This was the first vitamin to be discovered and isolated, which is why it is called B₁. A deficiency in B₁ causes a disease known as beriberi, which has been described for millennia. Beriberi is characterized by severe neurological and psychiatric symptoms (among other things) because the high energy demands of nerve and brain cells can't be met.

We have a limited ability to absorb thiamine, and while a frank deficiency is rare, levels decline quickly because we can't store this vitamin. Three modern factors have a great impact on thiamine levels: alcohol, high blood sugar, and exercise. Deficiency is common in people who drink too much alcohol, as it interferes with absorption in the intestine and decreases the storage of folate by the liver. High blood sugar and diabetes make you lose more thiamine in urine, and exercise increases your daily requirement. The need for thiamine also increases during more prolonged periods of increased energy demand, such as adolescent growth spurts, pregnancy, or lactation. Needs go up by 30 percent during pregnancy, and studies find that 25 to 40 percent of women have abnormally low levels.

Low thiamine presents with a host of symptoms: low energy, apathy, brain fog, irritability, and physical weakness.

AMOUNT YOU SHOULD EAT PER DAY: Women: 1.1mg / Men: 1.2 mg

INSUFFICIENT DIETARY INTAKE: 5–10% of US population. Higher in elderly; 30–50% of nursing home residents.

TOP 5 FOOD SOURCES: Pork (74% in 3 oz), sunflower seeds (43% in ¼ cup), trout (24% 3 oz), peas (19% in ½ cup), and pecans (17% in 1 oz)

TOP 5 RECIPES

1. Roasted Pork Loin and Red Cabbage–Fennel Sauerkraut = 107% (see page 212)
2. Pan-Roasted Duck with Cherry Sauce = 82% (see page 232)
3. Kale-Crusted Pork Chops = 81% (see page 209)
4. Chipotle Pork Loin with Blueberry-Kiwi Salsa = 76% (see page 221)
5. Cinnamon-Fennel Brined Pork Chops = 59% (see page 225)

COOKING EFFECT: B_1 is prone to damage from heat. Cooking reduces the vitamin B_1 content of food by roughly 20–50%.

ABSORPTION: Blocked by antithiamine factors in raw fish. Impaired by alcohol abuse.

STORAGE: Your body stores 30 mg, enough for 15–30 days.

Choline

Key to regulating anxiety, learning, and memory, choline is a cousin of the B vitamins. You use it to make phosphatidylcholine, the most common fat in all cells. It is needed to make the neurotransmitter acetylcholine, which is key to learning and memory. Choline also functions by donating methyl groups to the methylation cycle, much like the B vitamins. This cycle is a process fundamental to good energy, moods, and focus. Choline also regulates inflammation, and studies suggest it can help protect you from cognitive decline and dementia.

Choline is the most recent addition to the Institute of Medicine's "essential nutrients." While data indicate that people who consume more choline have lower levels of anxiety, the average American does not get nearly enough in his or her diet. Compounding this, about half of the US population has a specific genetic change that greatly increases the need for choline.

Choline is important for pregnant and breast-feeding women, as it is a critical vitamin during fetal development, particularly during the development of the brain, much like folate. Breast milk is very high in choline, and so breast-feeding mothers need a higher intake to prevent deficiency.

AMOUNT YOU SHOULD EAT PER DAY: Women: 425mg / Men: 550mg

INSUFFICIENT DIETARY INTAKE: 90% of US population

TOP 5 FOOD SOURCES: Beef liver (84% in 3 oz), eggs (35% in 1 egg), beef (22% in 3 oz), scallops (22% in 3 oz), and Brussels sprouts (15% in 1 cup)

TOP 5 RECIPES
1. Avocado Baked Egg = 69% (see page 124)
2. Deviled Green Eggs with Roasted Red Pepper = 69% (see page 153)
3. Cast-Iron Steak Dinner with Cauliflower = 68% (see page 218)
4. Whole Roasted Chicken with Anchovies and Olives = 68% (see page 210)
5. Truffled Farm Egg with Wilted Watercress = 45% (see page 123)

COOKING EFFECT: Choline appears to be fairly stable when heated or processed.

ABSORPTION: Celiac disease can affect absorption.

STORAGE: Your body stores are large, as this molecule is in every cell.

Calcium

Your body contains more calcium that any other mineral. While most often associated with bone health and recommended as a supplement to prevent osteoporosis, calcium plays a much more important role in your physiology: the communication between your brain cells requires this mineral. Each time one brain cell sends a message to another brain cell, calcium is used. The electricity pulsing through your neurons depends on it.

You likely already know that milk and dairy products are the main dietary sources of calcium. A surprising fact is that certain greens such as kale and bok choy possess highly absorbable forms of calcium as well. These greens have low levels of oxalates, which are the molecules in plants that bind tightly to calcium and prevent its absorption. In fact, a study found that more calcium was absorbed from kale than from milk, and on a per calorie basis it has higher concentrations.

Your absorption and use of calcium also depend on vitamin D, potassium, and magnesium, among other nutrients, so it should not be viewed in isolation.

AMOUNT YOU SHOULD EAT PER DAY: 1,000mg for women and men ages 31–50 / 1,200mg for women and men ages 51+

INSUFFICIENT DIETARY INTAKE: 73% of US population (43% of Americans take a calcium supplement)

TOP FOOD SOURCES: Yogurt (42% in 8 oz), cheese (31% in 1.5 oz), milk (30% in 8 oz), and kale (10% in 1 cup)

TOP 5 RECIPES
1. Crispy Shrimp with Greens and Beans = 49% (see page 257)
2. Kiwi Green Smoothie = 41% (see page 113)
3. Lazy Green Mac and Cheese = 40% (see page 162)
4. Millet-Cheddar Fritters = 33% (see page 138)
5. Citrus Scallops = 32% (see page 148)

COOKING EFFECT: Calcium is not affected by heat or storage.

ABSORPTION: Vitamin D improves calcium absorption, while oxalic acid and phytates in plants can decrease absorption (for example, spinach decreases the absorption of calcium when eaten together with kale or other calcium sources).

STORAGE: Calcium is the most common mineral in your body, making up 1.5 percent of your total mass (which equals one to two pounds for most people). High sodium, caffeine, protein, and alcohol intake can impair absorption, as can phosphorus and many processed foods. Proper absorbtion requires vitamin C, vitamin D, vitamin E, vitamin K, and magnesium.

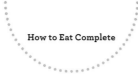

Potassium

With the advent of the Western diet, both the potassium: sodium ratio and the bicarbonate:chloride ratio have become reversed.

—Food and Nutrition Board, The Institute of Medicine

Every nerve impulse and each of your heartbeats depends on potassium. This mineral is highly concentrated inside your cells, which have about fifty times the concentration of potassium in your blood. Plants contain large amounts of potassium and calcium and very little sodium, which adds to the many reasons to eat a plant-based diet. In fact, the only way to get potassium is to eat more plants.

Humans have always eaten large amounts of potassium. Because of this dietary abundance, your kidneys are highly evolved to excrete potassium. This protects us against high potassium levels. Modern diets, however, are much lower in potassium. As we've consumed more processed foods, we've both decreased potassium and increased our intake of salt, sodium chloride. The balance of these minerals in our diet has essentially flip-flopped, leading to an intake that is incompatible with how your body works. Minerals such as potassium always travel with a partner that balances the mineral's charge. A diet that is low in potassium is also low in bicarbonate precursors that help balance the acidity in your blood. This sets off a cascade of events, because your body pulls calcium from bones to buffer your blood's acidity, leading to osteoporosis. Also, the kidneys attempt to retain calcium and this eventually leads to kidney stones. Low potassium intake and high sodium intake are also a main cause of high blood pressure, which damages the brain over time and leads to strokes.

AMOUNT YOU SHOULD EAT PER DAY: 4,700mg for women and men

INSUFFICIENT DIETARY INTAKE: 97% of US population

TOP 5 FOOD SOURCES: Beet greens (37% in 1 cup), Swiss chard (27% in 1 cup), spinach (24% in 1 cup), bananas (12% in 1 cup), and kale (8% in 1 cup)

TOP 5 RECIPES

1. Rainbow Burgers = 31% (see page 161)
2. Mussels with Garlicky Kale Ribbons = 30% (see page 239)
3. Summer Clam Chowder = 28% (see page 204)
4. Sunday Slow-Cooker Beef Shank = 28% (see page 230)
5. Pumpkin Soup with Macadamia Nuts = 27% (see page 191)

COOKING EFFECT: Boiling foods for a long time can cause a loss of potassium.

ABSORPTION: Caffeine can negatively affect potassium absorption.

STORAGE: 98% is stored inside cells. About 200mg per day is excreted in the urine. With no dietary intake, a mild deficiency develops in just 7 days.

Iodine

Iodine is key to the regulation of your metabolism, as its only role in the body is as an element of thyroid hormone. Without iodine, your metabolism slows, your energy drops, and the thyroid gland swells, producing a large fleshy mass called a goiter. This is commonplace in many developing countries and was quite common in the United States before the addition of iodine to table salt in the 1920s. Still, iodine intake dropped by about 50 percent in America from 1971 to 2000, and globally, 1.5 billion people are still deficient.

Increasing iodine intake does more than just prevent goiters; it also improves IQ and cognitive abilities. A lack of this mineral is the top cause of preventable mental retardation (a form called cretinism), as iodine is central to proper brain development. Thyroid hormone produced by the thyroid is 60 percent iodine and travels to the brain and plays a number of roles, such as assisting in the proper formation of myelin, the fatty insulation of brain cells. In recent years, there has been a clear public health message to reduce salt intake—causing potential problems if this is your only source of iodine. With iodine intake in the United States continuing to drop in the most recent 2010 NHANES by another 13 percent, and with levels in pregnant women quite low nationally, we need to get more iodine in our meals.

Seeking foods with a good dose of iodine leads us to seafood, a food group that is missing for so many people. Some sources, such as seaweed, are superconcentrated, as one gram of seaweed can contain 3,000 mcg. Iodine can also be found in products such as yogurt and milk, as well as the skin of potatoes.

Your iodine status is influenced by more than your intake. A number of new chemicals, such as flame-retardants (PBDEs) and brominated dough conditioners, contain bromine, which competes with iodine for uptake into the thyroid. There are also compounds called goitrogens found in plants (mostly in cruciferous vegetables, cassava, and soy) that can cause problems. For people with very low iodine intake, high intakes of these foods could be an issue. This does not mean you should banish Brussels sprouts and kale from your diet, but you should be mindful to increase your iodine intake from natural sources.

AMOUNT YOU SHOULD EAT PER DAY: 150mcg for women and men

INSUFFICIENT DIETARY INTAKE: 10% of US population. 37% of women ages 15–44; 56% of pregnant women. Worldwide: 30%.

TOP 5 FOOD SOURCES: Seaweed (500% in 1 tbsp), scallops (90% in 4 oz), cod (88% in 4 oz), yogurt (47% in 1 cup), and milk (38% in 8 oz)

TOP 6 RECIPES (AS THE LAST TWO CONTAIN THE SAME AMOUNT)
1. Citrus Scallops = 142% (see page 148)
2. Scallop-Shrimp Ceviche = 96% (see page 250)
3. Beet Greens with Homemade Citrus Wild Salmon Gravlax = 67% (see page 183)
4. Homemade Kefir with Apples = 59% (see page 127)

5. Avocado Baked Egg = 57% (see page 124)
6. Deviled Green Eggs with Roasted Red Pepper = 57% (see page 153)

COOKING EFFECT: Boiling causes losses of around 40%.

ABSORPTION: Iodine is rapidly absorbed.

STORAGE: Adults store 15–20mg of iodine, with about 70–80% stored in the thyroid gland.

Vitamin C

Vitamin C is a great team player—it lends electrons readily to other molecules, recharges your vitamin E, and eliminates the free radicals that age your brain and body. Ascorbic acid serves you in two main ways: as an antioxidant and as a cofactor in the biochemical reactions that create everything from the collagen in your skin to the brain chemicals that let you feel pleasure. Vitamin C is highly concentrated in the cerebral spinal fluid (CSF) that surrounds your brain, and higher levels of vitamin C in the CSF are associated with better cognitive performance as one ages.

Most mammals make vitamin C, but humans must eat it. Scurvy, a frank deficiency of vitamin C, is fatal. While you don't need much to prevent scurvy, just 10 milligrams a day, for optimal amounts you do need to focus on eating fruits and vegetables. Just two to three cups of the right plants per day will give you at least 200 milligrams, well above the RDA, but right in line with what nutrition researchers at the Linus Pauling Institute recommend. But almost half of all Americans don't even meet the RDA. The need for vitamin C goes up if you exercise heavily, are ill, or are under stress. Women who take oral birth control also need more vitamin C.

Vitamin C increases the absorption of iron, which is why adding lemon juice to everything from beans to oysters is smart.

AMOUNT YOU SHOULD EAT PER DAY: Women: 75mg / Men: 90 mg

INSUFFICIENT DIETARY INTAKE: 48% of US population

TOP 5 FOOD SOURCES: Papaya (224% in 1 medium fruit), bell peppers (157% in 1 cup), broccoli (135% in 1 cup), Brussels sprouts (125% in 1 cup), and strawberries (113% in 1 cup)

TOP 5 RECIPES

1. Kiwi Green Smoothie = 260% (see page 113)
2. Country Ribs with Millet = 249% (see page 222)
3. Pancetta Brussels Sprouts = 187% (see page 151)
4. Whole Roasted Chicken with Anchovies and Olives = 179% (see page 210)
5. Buttermilk Strawberry Smoothie = 172% (see page 117)

COOKING EFFECT: Baking, broiling, and panfrying lower the content of vitamin C, but boiling lowers it even further.

ABSORPTION: 70–90% of vitamin C in foods is absorbed at moderate intakes (up to 130mg a day). Doses above 1g per day cause absorption to fall to 50% as you only saturate your transporters.

STORAGE: Your body doesn't store vitamin C, so you need a continuous supply.

The *Eat Complete* Essential 21 Nutrients

NUTRIENT	RDA MEN/WOMEN	AMOUNT STORED
7 FOR FOUNDATION		
OMEGA-3 FATS (DHA/EPA AND ALA)	DHA/EPA: 500mg (no RDA; amount based on international recommendations) ALA: 1.6g/1.1g	Stored in the body
ZINC	11mg/8mg	Not stored in the body
VITAMIN B$_{12}$ (COBALAMIN)	2. 4mcg	2–3 years' worth
MAGNESIUM	420mg/350mg	25mg
VITAMIN B$_9$ (FOLATE)	400mcg	10–30mg
FIBER AND PROBIOTICS	Fiber: 38mg/25mg. Probiotics: No established RDA	Fiber: Body does not store. Probiotics: The gut contains trillions of bacteria.
COMPLETE PROTEINS	56g/46g	Makes up 20% of your body mass, mostly in the muscle
7 FOR PROTECTION		
VITAMIN E	15mg	Not stored as readily as other fat soluble vitamins
VITAMIN K	120mcg/90mcg	Limited capacity for storage
VITAMIN A AND CAROTENOIDS	900mcg/700mcg	Dependent on intake

SYMPTOMS OF DEFICIENCY	PERCENTAGE IN THE US WITH INSUFFICIENT DIETARY INTAKE	TOP FOOD SOURCES
Poor focus and memory, low mood, anxiety, accelerated brain aging	98%, estimated; no established information	DHA/EPA: Fish oil, salmon, herring, mackerel, tuna ALA: Flaxseed oil, chia seeds, walnuts, canola oil, navy beans
Frequent infections, loss of hair, poor appetite, skin sores, problems with sense of taste and smell	42%	Oysters, steak, sesame seeds, pumpkin seeds, ground turkey
Fatigue, brain fog, anemia, muscle weakness, hypotension, mood disturbances	20%; 73% of vegans have deficient or insufficient blood levels	Clams, beef liver, mussels, sardines, crab, trout, wild salmon
Weak bones, loss of appetite, nausea, vomiting, retention of sodium, anxiety	68%	Almonds, spinach, cashews, black beans, soybeans
Depression, anxiety, anemia, fatigue, gray hair, mouth sores	75%	Chicken liver, lentils, chickpeas, black-eyed peas, Brussels sprouts, asparagus, cooked spinach
Fiber: Constipation, weight gain, nausea, fatigue Probiotics: Poor digestive health, impaired immunity, depression	Fiber: 97% Probiotics: No established information	Fiber: Navy beans, lentils, tempeh, raspberries, collard greens Probiotics: Yogurt, kefir, sauerkraut, kombucha
Mood changes, hunger, thinning hair, weakness, trouble focusing, impaired immunity	8% of girls and women	Animal sources: Turkey, salmon, beef, chicken, tuna Plant sources: Soybeans, lentils, white beans, peas, kidney beans
Weakness, loss of coordination, hemolytic anemia	96%	Sunflower seeds, almonds, spinach, avocado, olive oil
Easy bruising, bloody gums, heavy menstruation, osteoporosis, osteoarthritis	75%	Kale, spinach, mustard greens, collard greens, beet greens
Night blindness, dry skin	40% men; 32% women	Sweet potato, carrots, pumpkin, chicken liver, mustard greens

NUTRIENT	RDA MEN/WOMEN	AMOUNT STORED
PHYTONUTRIENTS	No RDA	Not stored in the body
MONOUNSATURATED FATS (MUFAS)	No RDA	Stored in the body
VITAMIN D	15mcg	Stores vary widely depending on sun exposure and intake
SELENIUM	55mcg	Not stored in the body

7 FOR IGNITION

IRON	8mg/18mg	3.5g
VITAMIN B$_1$ (THIAMINE)	1.2mg/1.1mg	30mg
CHOLINE	550mg/425mg	Large stores in the body
CALCIUM	1,000mg (ages 31–50) /1,200mg (ages 51+)	Mostly stored in the bones and teeth; most common mineral in the body
POTASSIUM	4,700mg	120g; mostly stored inside the body's cells
IODINE	150 mcg	15–20mg
VITAMIN C	90mg/75mg	Not stored in the body

SYMPTOMS OF DEFICIENCY	PERCENTAGE IN THE US WITH INSUFFICIENT DIETARY INTAKE	TOP FOOD SOURCES
Low energy, weight gain, low mood	80%	Dark chocolate, blueberries, hazelnuts, artichokes
Fatigue, high blood cholesterol, depression	80%, estimated; no established information	Macadamia nuts, almonds, peanuts, avocado, olive oil
Fatigue, muscle aches and weakness, osteoporosis, high blood pressure, cardiovascular disease, depression	85–90%; deficiency is very common	Wild salmon, trout, sardines, tuna, pork ribs, eggs
Male infertility, hypothyroidism	15%	Brazil nuts, lobster, tuna, shrimp, halibut
Weakness and fatigue, cognitive fog, low mood, dizziness, and cold hands/feet	20%; more common in vegetarians and vegans; women are more likely to be deficient	Soybeans, oysters, dark chocolate, sesame seeds, spinach
Fatigue, poor memory, irritability, loss of appetite, weight loss. Severe deficiency is known as beriberi and can cause nerve, heart, and brain abnormalities.	5–10%; higher in elderly	Pork, sunflower seeds, trout, peas, pecans
Fatigue, insomnia, learning problems	90%; many people of all ages are at risk for deficiency	Beef liver, eggs, beef, scallops, Brussels sprouts
Numbness, muscle cramps, lethargy, osteoporosis	73%	Yogurt, cheese, milk, kale
Constipation, fatigue, muscle weakness, numbness	97%	Beet greens, Swiss chard, spinach, bananas, kale
Hypothyroidism, goiter, growth and developmental abnormalities	10%; 50% pregnant women	Seaweed, scallops, cod, yogurt, milk
Weakness, irritability, fatigue. In its severe form, can lead to scurvy.	48%	Papaya, bell peppers, broccoli, Brussels sprouts, strawberries

Your Food Prescription
ASSESSMENT AND
ACTION PLAN

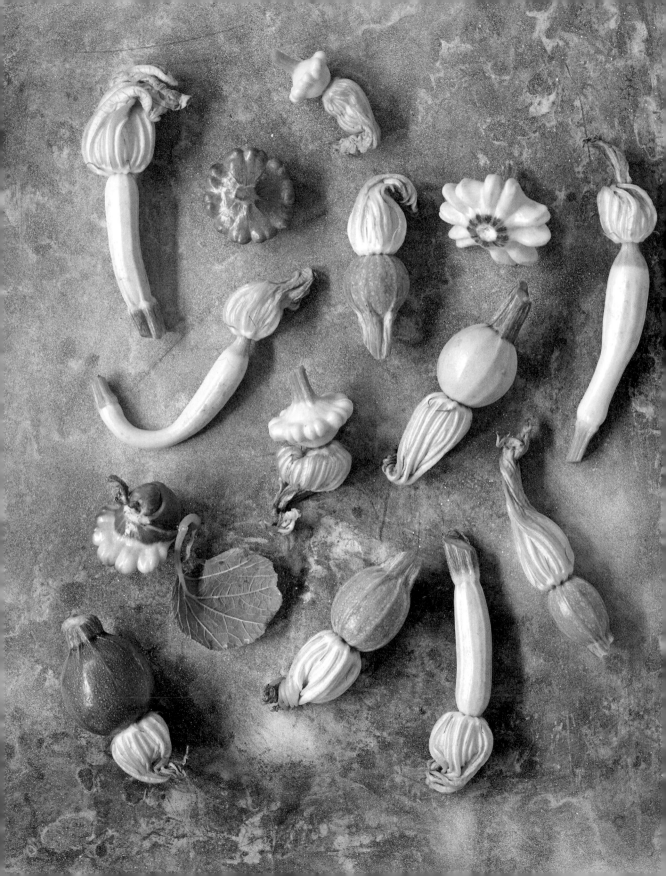

nderstanding your food habits, both good and bad, is the first step to transforming your health with food. Honest assessment allows you to best plan a food intervention and create strategies to easily incorporate any missing foods and nutrients. Little changes do lead to big changes, and I often tell my patients that "the best step is the next step."

While reviewing the diet of a young graduate student who I treat for anxiety and depression, I mentioned that nuts make a great snack. He made a face that clearly said "yuck." As it turned out, he had tried nuts only a few times in his life, and perhaps not since he was about six years old. Nuts tasted "waxy" to him and he didn't like the mouthfeel.

I happened to have a bag of raw almonds and cashews in my office and invited him to try a few. I wondered if he had eaten roasted nuts in the past and I thought perhaps a raw nut would not have a waxy mouthfeel to him. I asked him first to just put an almond in his month and suck on it before chewing it, a mini mindful eating exercise. He sheepishly admitted that he had never eaten a cashew before.

This small experiment completely shifted my patient's dietary pattern. He found that nibbling on nuts was a great replacement for the candies and chips he would normally eat while studying. "I love nuts now—I probably eat three ounces a day," he told me when I saw him a few weeks later.

This patient also disliked seafood, but again, it was mainly out of inexperience and limited exposure. He told me his family never ate fish when he was growing up, or if they did it was fish sticks. Over the following months, he started cooking a bit more, first to impress his girlfriend, and then as a bit of a challenge to himself to eat better and expand his palate. It was all done in small steps: a bite of sushi, trying his hand at fish tacos, and even sampling his first oyster. He didn't like everything, of course, but what struck me as his physician was that a simple focus on trying new foods could radically shift his dietary pattern. Adding nuts gave him more minerals, MUFAs, and phytonutrients, all helpful to brain health, and replaced his candy snacks that both made him feel guilty and provided no brain nutrients.

I developed a food assessment in my practice with the goal of getting a broad view of what my patients eat on a regular basis. After all, it is not the occasional slice of birthday cake or once-a-year Christmas ham that really has an impact on our health. We are most influenced by the foods we eat on a daily and weekly basis.

Maybe your dietary pattern doesn't need a complete overhaul. But even if it does, changing your food choices happens one meal at a time. Adding single foods from previously unconsidered food groups can greatly enhance the nutritional value of your meals. In my clinical practice, there is no room for dietary affiliations—meaning that whether you are a dedicated Paleo eater or a vegan, my role is to help you feed your brain within your personal eating philosophy.

The Simple Food Assessment

Food can get complicated, and I want to keep things simple—so I call this the Simple Food Assessment. This assessment will allow you to understand more about your dietary pattern, which will help you see some gaps and places for change. Often people already know where they need to improve. Trust this intuition.

A patient of mine was hooked on diet soda and would drink at least six 20-ounce bottles a day before 4:00 p.m. It didn't take complex diagnostics to see where the problem was. He knew this was an issue that needed to be fixed, but he liked sipping on something throughout the day. Talking through the healthier options such as coffee and tea, or even infused water, helped him shift towards healthier choices. One day he showed up with a cup of coffee. Today, he drinks only a few diet sodas a week.

Let's take a few minutes now to think about your dietary pattern, your challenges, and your goals. I find that assessing food is best done by walking through your day. We'll start with the details of what you tend to eat for each meal of the day. Since we are looking for patterns, think more of the foods you eat regularly than the outliers. Then identify some challenges you have for each meal. Finally, let's set some concrete achievable goals.

For example, in our house, most days start with some fruit, usually berries or melon, and a cup of coffee with grass-fed whole milk followed by eggs, oatmeal or yogurt with nuts and seeds, or a smoothie. That's our pattern. There is a nice mix of proteins, fats, and carbohydrates, mostly plant-based foods, and lots of colors. I feel pretty good about breakfast, but I have a few challenges. I sometimes skip breakfast, and, if I am being honest, my smoothies have just been fruits and nuts lately because I keep forgetting to buy kefir. My goals for this week are to eat at least a piece of fruit or an egg with my coffee every morning even if I am in a rush (I'll hard-boil six eggs on Sunday), and to buy kefir.

The following pages will help you understand your pattern, get a clear sense of your challenges, and set some short-term goals. Writing things down helps us think about them differently. A few words about goals—make them small and specific. Instead of a goal like "eat healthier this week," focus on specific foods or nutrients you need. Do you see that your pattern is missing seafood? Eat wild salmon this week. Specific, short-term goals are more likely to be enacted. Focus on complete eating one meal at a time.

Food Allergies

The list of top food allergies contains many of the most important brain foods: nuts, eggs, and shellfish. Food allergies range from mild rashes and gut distress (bloating, pain, bowel problems) to full anaphylactic shock, which can be fatal. If you have a food allergy or begin to develop one, make sure you work with a health care provider to have an action plan, and, if needed, an epinephrine autoinjector or EpiPen. Often, food allergies are fairly specific—a person can have an allergy to cashews but not to almonds. If you need to cut out specific core *Eat Complete* foods, make a list of the essential 21 nutrients in that food and swap in other foods with those nutrients to replace them.

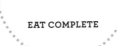

Eat Complete Breakfast

What do you eat for breakfast? _____

Breakfast Challenges _____

Breakfast Goals _____

Eat Complete Lunch

What do you eat for lunch? _____

Lunch Challenges _____

Lunch Goals _____

Eat Complete Dinner

What do you eat for dinner? _____

Dinner Challenges _____

Dinner Goals _____

- Do you have regular snacks or eat at other times of the day?
- What are the religious, cultural, or moral rules that influence your eating?
- Do you have any food allergies?
- Do you have any food aversions or foods you avoid?
- What is your favorite meal?
- Are there any foods you crave?

* How often do you cook at home?

* When and where do you eat out?

* When and where do you shop for food?

* My Rainbow. List your favorite fruits and vegetables:

    Red: _____

    Orange: _____

    Yellow: _____

    Green: _____

    Blue/Purple: _____

    White: _____

Breakfast

This meal really sets the tone for the day. To start the day "eating complete" requires some smart planning and execution. Given the epidemic of sleep deprivation, mornings can be tough. Breakfast needs to be simple, easy to clean up, and satisfying.

The breakfast recipes in *Eat Complete* fall into four categories: egg dishes, smoothies, yogurt, and baked goods. Diversity in your morning routine ensures you start your day a bit more curious and inspired, while also ensuring you get a variety of different nutrients day to day. Most people tend to eat a relatively high-carbohydrate, low-fat, and low-protein meal in the mornings, such as breakfast cereal and low-fat milk, which usually leads to a bout of mid-morning hunger. Another

problem can be getting a rainbow of colors. I favor breakfasts that contain all three macronutrients: carbohydrates, protein, and fats. These, along with some fiber, help keep you satiated until lunch.

Common Breakfast Problems

* No breakfast at all or a rushed breakfast.
* A meal of mainly sugar and simple carbs: pancakes, muffins, bagels, toast, and breakfast cereal.
* Lack of diversity in breakfast choices.
* No plant-based proteins such as beans, nuts, or greens.
* No seafood.
* No rainbow vegetables or leafy greens.
* Conventional dairy instead of grass-fed.
* Use of skim milk.
* Low-quality eggs.

- No MUFAs or PUFAs, which are usually found in olive oil and seafood.
  - Low-quality meat choices, such as nitrate-laden, extra-salty bacon.
  - Use of premade foods such as frozen hash browns instead of a real potato.

Lunch

Lunch keeps your motor running . . . or not. With a natural second peak of the "sleep" hormone melatonin at 3 p.m., the wrong lunch choices can leave you nodding off instead of plowing through.

Since lunch is a meal often eaten out of the home, the challenge to *Eat Complete* can seem formidable. Tempting, delicious, and convenient, fast food feels like all we can cram into the brief time we allow for lunch. There are two common problems I see with lunch. The first is sourcing: what are the healthiest, best-value options for days when you don't bring your lunch? We take for granted that lunch has to be a rushed, nonorganic meal, but options exist. Second is the habit of not bringing your own lunch. Years ago when I was a resident, an older psychoanalyst supervised my work. He would eat a turkey sandwich loaded with avocados, tomatoes, and greens while he listened to my notes and questions. It was a healthy option, and he also saved

money. "Bringing my lunch put my kids through college," he told me one day. He also ate slowly and thoughtfully, all while getting some light work done. Deli meat, even turkey, isn't a great choice, but he loaded up on the plants and used high-quality whole grain bread.

Many of the small plates and salads in this book are easy to pack in jars and make for a great midday meal. Other options are to pack a smoothie or to use the leftovers from a main dish such as the Grilled Wild Salmon with Garlic Scape Pesto and Summer Squash on page 245 or the Cinnamon-Fennel Brined Pork Chop with Cauliflower Hash on page 225 and put them over lightly dressed greens. To avoid the slump, avoid both large meals and simple sugars as both make you sleepier. Remember to transition your body from working mode to eating mode. Lunch is time to recharge and get ready for round two of the day.

Common Lunch Problems

- No actual break from work to eat.
- Rushed eating due to anxiety, leading to little chewing and to "wolfing down" food.
- A meal of mindless meat and simple carbs: burger and fries, tacos, and pepperoni pizza.
- Reliance on restaurants and fast food.
- Low-nutrient-dense greens such as iceberg lettuce as the salad base.

- Low-quality deli meats such as ham, salami, or flavored meats like BBQ chicken tenders.
  - Early-afternoon fatigue due to wrong food choices and excess food.
  - No seafood.
  - Sugary beverages, especially non-sodas that still provide a giant dose of sugar: iced teas, fruit smoothies, and energy drinks.
  - No equipment or plan to bring your food. (Try jars, a lunch box, or a thermos.)
  - No smart treat options. (Try a little dark chocolate, a coffee or tea with milk, or a piece of fruit such as an apple.)
  - No snack stash. (Keep good-quality snacks at your workplace: dried fruit, nuts, cheese, dark chocolate or dark chocolate–covered coffee beans or almonds. Stress eating happens, so use something good for you instead of junk from a vending machine.)

Dinner

The last meal of the day is an opportunity to fill in any nutrient gaps and to settle down and digest the day. Arriving home after a stressful day to an empty fridge and no plan for dinner can easily lead to going out or ordering in—and making poor food choices while hungry.

Instead, arrive home to a few light snacks, maybe the Clove-Spiked Cocktail Nut Mix on page 144 or the Creamy Marsala Wine Pâté on page 143. Then mix up your protein source—I recommend starting with two seafood dinners and two vegetarian dinners per week as a good guide.

Don't make the mistake of thinking dinner has to be complicated. Scrambled eggs and vegetables can be a quick, nutrient-dense meal. Leftovers make a great base. Recently, I had one head of cabbage and one leftover pork chop, which in a few minutes became a great meal for our family. Many of the recipes have notes about batch cooking. In our freezer we have jars of cooked grains, lentils, and beans, and metal ice cube trays we fill with stock (see page 200). With just a few minutes of defrosting, usually while we make a simple salad, we sit down to something home-cooked.

Common Dinner Problems

- No advance planning. (Keep it simple: Plan. Shop. Cook.)
- Dread of dishes. (Cook neatly and be clean.)
- No appetizer course. (Transition from work or school to home with a snack.)
- Habituation to a pattern of meat, vegetable, and starch. (Think about plant-

based dishes, using meat as your protein only a few nights a week.)

❀ Lack of variety of flavors and protein sources. (Experiment with fresh herbs, new spices such as turmeric, and more seafood.)

❀ Rainbow vegetables only in the salad. (Use them as sides and mix up raw and cooked.)

❀ Reliance on refined white carbohydrates such as pasta and white rice. (Use whole grains, and not just whole grain flours— think wheat berry, quinoa, and brown rice.)

❀ Need for more diverse seafood choices. (Go with wild seafood and use creative ways such as adding anchovies in salad dressings.)

❀ Too much alcohol. (People get into the habit of daily drinking. This is often because alcohol is so calming. Deal with stress using exercise and mindful breathing instead. Try kombucha, herbal teas, and water as alternatives.)

❀ Eating in front of the TV or another screen. (Try to unplug during meals.)

Food Fixes

Food assessment and prescription is a very individual process, but there are a number of patterns that tend to emerge in my clinical practice. There are the people who eat a "beige diet" lacking in plants and colors, and there are others who don't eat

much seafood at all. Many are too busy to cook or shop. Following are some of the most common food concerns and my best tips for addressing each issue, paired with recipes from the book.

Leafy Greens

Dark greens such as kale taste bitter.
About 15 percent of people are "supertasters" and are particularly sensitive to the bitter compounds in greens. For some, the bitterness can be mellowed by cooking the greens: for example, sautéing them with onions. Try using baby greens instead of adult greens. Another option is to eat these greens in late fall after the frost, which is when greens such as kale tend to sweeten. The molecules that cause bitterness are different in various greens, so experiment a bit to find the best choice for you. Bok choy, mesclun, purslane, beet greens, watercress, and red cabbage are milder to some eaters, and they provide nutrients similar to those found in the more boldly flavored kale and mustard greens.

Vegetables

Organic is too expensive.
By eating seasonally and getting more food from a local farmers' market, you can eat organic foods without breaking the bank. Join a Community Supported Agriculture (CSA) program for both amazing value and exposure to new vegetables. Freeze, can,

or ferment your extras from the bounty of the summer. Frozen organic vegetables are a good value and equivalent to fresh vegetables in terms of nutrients. Remember that organic matters more for some foods, such as kale and peaches (which are eaten whole), than others, such as onions and sweet potatoes (which are peeled). Use the Environmental Working Groups list of the Dirty Dozen and Clean Fifteen as a guide to making informed decisions about produce. You can also ask your local farmers (if possible) about their produce, as many small farms aren't officially certified organic but still grow food free of pesticides. Finally, many states offer matching programs that make food stamps worth double their value at farmers' markets.

Nuts

Nuts have too many calories.

The USDA issued a statement in 2015 that the caloric guidance on nuts overestimates the calories they contain by about 25 percent. Nuts and seeds are great snacks, as they contain health-promoting MUFA and PUFA fats, provide minerals like zinc and magnesium that promote brain growth, and are the top source of vitamin E, which protects brain fat.

I eat too many nuts.

Make sure to buy your nuts raw and unsalted. Excess salt makes you eat more nuts, so flavor and roast them yourself.

Dairy

I am lactose intolerant.

Using fermented dairy such as kefir eliminates most of the lactose. If you are very sensitive you can find most fermented dairy products in lactose-free forms. Aged cheeses also tend to be very low in lactose.

I eat a low-fat, flavored yogurt every morning.

Yogurt is a great start to the day, but many yogurts are small containers of excess sugar. This is especially true of low-fat and nonfat flavored yogurts. You get better value and more control by purchasing plain yogurt and flavoring it yourself with fresh fruit and berries, nuts, and honey. You can also add needed morning nutrients like fiber to keep you full by adding in toppings such as pumpkin or chia seeds.

Meat

Eating meat is unhealthy, unethical, and cruel, plus it destroys the environment.

The merits of meat will continue to be debated. As a former long-term vegetarian, I believe it is possible to eat meat in a healthy, responsible, and sustainable way. In terms of health, the goal of *Eat Complete* is to help you eat meat more mindfully. The animals I've seen raised on pastures in small farms produce a meat that is much lower in the two factors considered unhealthy: saturated fat and cholesterol. Also, these animals have very good lives. But eating a diet with excess meat is bad for the environment and eating meat of any kind does increase your environmental impact. Choose meat from smaller farms that are well managed for a better-quality meat that keeps your food dollars local.

Grass-fed, local meat costs too much. Using low-cost cuts such as the shank and liver and taking part in a meat share by buying a larger quantity are two strategies that save money. Some Community Supported Agriculture (CSA) programs offer an option to include meat. Some of the extra cost might be worth it to you. Realistically, grass-fed beef should cost a bit more as you get a healthier food that provides more nutrients. Spending a bit more on local meat also pays you back in a number of ways, such as providing jobs in your community.

Eggs

Eggs have too much cholesterol. Dietary cholesterol does not appear to be much of a risk factor in health. You don't absorb the majority of cholesterol that you eat, and for most people, dietary cholesterol doesn't have much of an effect on the numbers of your cholesterol profile that your doctor checks.

I don't know which eggs to buy. Eggs range greatly in price and less so in nutritional quality. Ideally, get your eggs from a small farmer who lets the birds roam wild. These are the most nutrient-dense eggs. Otherwise, get the best eggs you can afford. I think the extra dollar for a dozen organic, pasture-raised, or cage-free eggs is worth it. The omega-3 fats advertised on cartons are usually shorter-chained ALA as the birds are generally fed flax, and so are not a good source of longer-chained omega-3s. But eggs of almost any price are great value nutritionally.

Do colored eggs have more nutrients? Eggs from some chickens are hues of blue and green. Choosing these eggs doesn't change much nutritionally, but you support diversity in the population of egg layers and reward farmers who try something different.

Seafood

All seafood tastes fishy to me. Because seafood contains more PUFAs than other meat, it can spoil more quickly. Fresh seafood won't smell or taste fishy, though some fresh seafood such as mackerel and anchovy has a stronger taste than milder fish such as wild salmon or trout. Start with milder fish and with dishes that are more strongly flavored, such as the Garlic Butter Shrimp over Spiralized Zucchini on page 246 or the Rocket Pie on 237. Begin with small amounts and give your palate time to adjust. Another mild option is the Citrus Scallops with Spinach, Asparagus, and Marinated Kirby Cucumber on page 148.

I'm worried about getting too much mercury.

Don't eat fish that have high amounts of mercury. Just avoid shark, swordfish, tilefish, and king mackerel and limit albacore tuna to six ounces or less per week. Concerns about mercury have limited seafood intake by pregnant women, prompting the EPA and FDA to issue a statement encouraging pregnant women to eat seafood two or three times per week. In general you get little to no mercury in smaller fish such as anchovies and bivalves such as mussels.

I don't know which fish to buy.

Two resources make buying easy. First, check out an online guide—such as the Monterey Bay Aquarium's Seafood Watch guide and app—that rates fish according to factors like sustainability. Second, get to know your fishmonger. Ask what is fresh. Tell him or her what you like and get some advice.

Beans and Legumes

Beans give me too much gas.

Soak beans in warm water with a little vinegar for 12 to 24 hours and change the water a few times. This is easy to do in a slow cooker. Eat smaller quantities of beans, and don't mix with other foods that often cause gas such as Brussels sprouts. Other helpful tricks are to chew more, and to add more fermented foods to your diet. Over time, eating more plants helps populate your gut with bugs that better digest beans.

I don't like the starchy taste of beans.

Use beans in hummus or other blended dips. Try smaller beans and legumes such as lentils and small red beans.

Spices

"Healthy" food doesn't taste very good to me.

Spices are unheralded sources of nutrients. If you have been on a steady diet of highly processed food with artificial flavorings, spices and herbs will be key as you transition back to the world of natural flavors. Spices and herbs have more antioxidant power per weight than any other food group. You should upgrade by replacing unused old spices, which lose flavor over time. Many spices are most aromatic and flavorful when combined with fats that also help emulsify the spices and spread them over the dish. Fresh is more flavorful, so when possible use fresh herbs in place of dried. We'll cover this in more detail in the next chapter.

Beverages

I get all my fruits and vegetables in juice.

Eating whole fruits and vegetables is preferable to drinking juice. An orange will always trump orange juice. While juicing can seem as if you are extracting the essence of the plant, you leave behind much of the fiber, which keeps you full and slows down the digestion of sugars. You also end up taking in a larger bolus of sugar much faster than by consuming fruits and veggies whole.

Our household is hooked on soda.

With 35 grams of sugar per 12 ounces and no nutrients for the brain, soda is still a staple for many people even though consumption is dropping. The average teenage boy in America still gets about 20 percent of his daily calories from soda. Soda can be swapped out for sweetened herbal teas, juice mixed with seltzer, or fermented drinks such as kombucha (which can contain small amounts of alcohol).

I know red wine is healthy so I drink it every day.

Red wine contains some high concentrations of phytonutrients such as tannins that appear to protect and relax arteries, which helps preserve blood flow to the brain. One of wine's phytonutrients, resveratrol, gained much attention after high doses were shown to prolong life in animal models. Resveratrol is not highly absorbed. Red wine is a staple of the Mediterranean diet and some health

benefits are associated with moderate wine consumption. However, alcohol is easy to overconsume and wine is often an overlooked source of simple sugars and calories that can drive hunger. For people who struggle with low moods, energy, or focus, daily wine isn't a good idea. After all, alcohol is classified medically as a central nervous system depressant.

I drink coffee daily and tea rarely.

Just as eating the rainbow of vegetables gives you a mix of healing plant-based compounds, drinking a variety of teas seems to have a number of health benefits. Try alternating your daily jolt of joe with black tea. Or use herbal teas to replace sugary beverages. Tea is also a great way to deliver health-promoting phytonutrients to kids.

The ritual of tea, a time to settle and reflect, exists in many cultures for good reason. Life is richer with a moment of reflection. Fermenting tea for two weeks yields kombucha, a fizzy, complex brew, which is a good source of probiotic "good bugs" and another way to get the benefits of tea's polyphenols. Be aware that kombucha often has a small amount of alcohol.

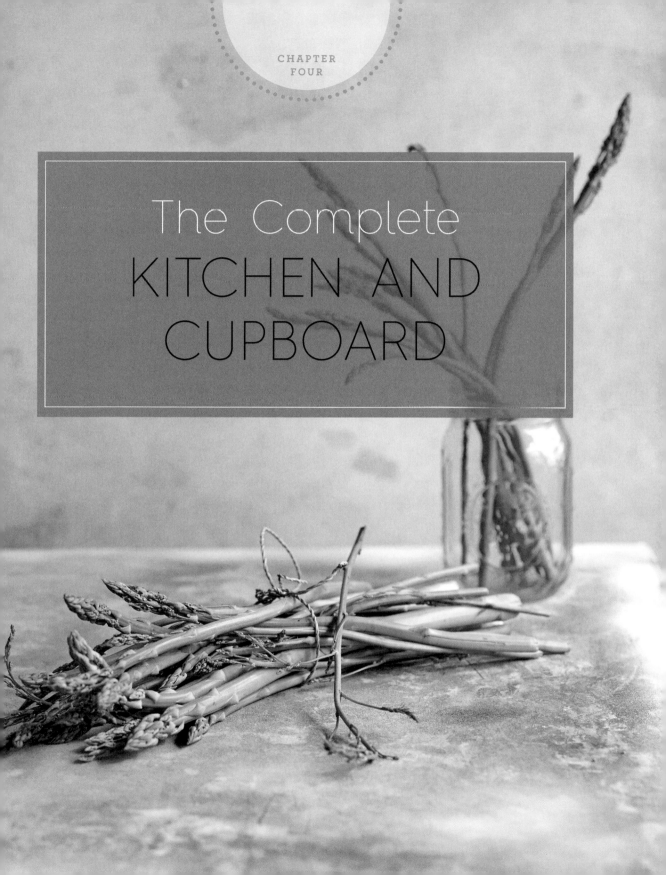

The Complete
KITCHEN AND
CUPBOARD

This chapter is a quick guide to the tools, spices, and techniques that are used in the recipes that follow. The primary idea is to put you in control of your food by making cooking basic and feasible. Most recipes will require only a knife, a zester, an iron skillet, and inspiration. Spices and herbs, along with their overlooked health benefits, will be highlighted, in features on turmeric, rosemary, mint, edible flowers, etc. The cooking fats—olive oil, coconut oil, and butter—will be presented along with their nutritional attributes and cooking roles.

There are many good reasons people don't eat complete. Often there's not enough time or money. Sometimes it's a lack of experience in the kitchen. Who likes doing the dishes anyway?

The focus of this chapter is to help you save money and use your time efficiently in the kitchen. Some of the ingredients in this book may be new to you, so let's give them a proper introduction highlighting the delicious flavors and important nutrients they yield. Let's also make sure your kitchen is stocked with the needed tools and equipment to pull off all the recipes in *Eat Complete*. And then there is the issue of confidence: many people I meet are quite convinced that they cannot cook. If that is you, I'd invite you to consider another possibility.

I remember when we first moved to New York City. I was twenty-six, pushing through my intern year at Columbia University Medical Center and New York-Presbyterian Hospital. Back then I was transitioning out of being a vegetarian. Based on the research I was reading about omega-3 fats, I knew I wanted to eat more seafood. I faced two significant barriers, however: I didn't like fish and I couldn't cook fish.

I offered this up one night to a chef I'd met. "Oh it's so easy," she exclaimed. "Get a nice mild white fish, top it with a few pats of butter and lemon zest, and heat your oven to three fifty. Cook the fish for eight minutes and then turn on the broiler for a minute or two. Take it out, and if the flesh separates, it's done." I was terrified of undercooked seafood, but this struck me as pretty simple.

The next night I stopped by the market and bought some flounder for dinner. It was easy to prepare, and while it was not my favorite meal, it was a first step. Over the following years, I explored more seafood, adding in salmon, building my way up to mackerel (after a tip from a Malaysian man to top it with lots of ginger), and on to today, when I regularly shuck oysters and steam mussels at home.

All of this is to say that with a few basic tools, some herbs and spices, fresh ingredients, and a basic desire, you can cook anything. These fundamentals are what help me eat complete in my own kitchen.

Gluten-Free Grains

Get more grain diversity to get a more diverse set of nutrients and phytonutrients. As I mentioned in the *Eat Complete* principles, I don't think that gluten is unhealthy for most people—but this book is mainly gluten-free to show the many different options of grain available to you. Grains are appealing as they are easy to store, nutrient dense, and inexpensive. They are also a surprising source of phytonutrients. Swapping simple sugars and refined carbohydrates found in most processed foods and baked goods for more complex carbohydrates like those in whole grains could be the single most important step for many of you reading this. Some professionals feel that simple carbs are "addictive," and many of my patients certainly report being helpless to resist. (Occasionally, I must have toast.) But getting rid of the fast, simple sugars and moving to the more complex, slowly digested carbohydrates is key as you can satisfy a craving for carbs without a shock to the system. Plus you just get more nutrients. Simply swapping white rice for brown rice or even black rice makes a big difference.

RICE. This seed of grass is a staple around the world. The practice of "polishing" rice by removing the outer layer in order to refine it led to the discovery of the first vitamin, thiamine. Removing this layer stripped all the thiamine and led to beriberi, a disease of weakness, mood and memory disturbances, and eventually irreversible brain damage.

Brown, wild, and black rice all have

more nutrient density and more interesting flavor profiles. Leaving on the outer layer means you get a slower-digesting, healthier carbohydrate. Upgrading your rice might be aided by getting a rice cooker.

MILLET. This small grain is the sixth most consumed worldwide. There are many varieties: pearl, finger, and foxtail. In general, millet contains more protein and fiber than most grains. It has 50 percent more protein than brown rice and three times more iron than wheat. It is an excellent source of magnesium. Foxtail millet contains ten times more calcium than other millets or grains. Millet is also known for having a high concentration of polyphenols, the family of phytonutrients linked to better heart health, lower rates of diabetes, and anticancer effects. Highly drought-resistant, millet is a good source of nutrition in arid regions. Before rice became the staple of China, millet was the dominant grain.

TEFF. Indigenous to Ethiopia, this is one of the original grains cultivated by humans. It is small, about the size of a poppy seed, and still used to make *injera*, a traditional Ethiopian spongy flat bread. Teff contains a very high-quality protein and is an excellent source of fiber.

AMARANTH. This pseudocereal grain was the staple of food for the ancient Aztecs.

It is high in protein and a good source of the essential amino acid lysine, which is missing from many grains and corn. It is high in magnesium, iron, and calcium. It contains a number of phytonutrients under investigation for their anti-inflammatory and anticancer effects.

QUINOA. The United Nations declared 2013 the year of quinoa. A pseudocereal like amaranth, quinoa is fast to prepare and it possesses a high-quality protein. It has more MUFAs than most grains and a very deep bench of nutrients with good concentrations of magnesium, vitamin E, fiber, folate, and zinc. Quinoa also has high amounts of phytonutrients, and some varieties have as many polyphenols as berries.

Beans and Legumes

Dried beans and legumes offer some of the best nutritional value in the grocery store. A few dollars will purchase a pound of dried beans and legumes—an amazing value compared with canned beans. Increasing your use of lentils, beans, and chickpeas is an important source of more plant-based protein, minerals, and essential B vitamins in your diet. For example, a cup

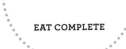
of lentils contains 90 percent of your daily need of folate. Beans are also very high in polyphenol antioxidants—in fact, the top-rated food in terms of sheer antioxidant power is small, red beans, which top even blueberries.

Herbs

Cooking with fresh herbs is a mainstay for restaurant chefs and accomplished home cooks alike. If you haven't had your hands on the fresh stuff yet, get ready for some serious flavor from very little effort. Most of the recipes provide ideas on which herbs pair well with which proteins and spices, but I'm also including some ideas here to help inspire experimentation.

BASIL pairs well with veggies and fruits that have a high water content, such as fresh tomatoes, zucchini, and watermelon. Use it with mild proteins such as white fish, chicken, and shrimp. It is delectable with soft and hard cheeses alike, such as goat cheese, feta, mozzarella, and Parmesan. Basil comes in many varieties, from Italian (sweet mint and anise), to Sweet Thai (a hint of pepper), to Dark Opal (similar in taste to Italian but deep purple in color).

CHIVES, a type of onion, have a mild flavor that pairs well with any ingredient that needs a hint of onion. Sprinkle them over fish, both smoked and fresh, or use them with a wide range of vegetables from artichokes to zucchini. Chives are especially good in delicate sauces made with a sprinkle of Parmesan or a crumble of fresh farm cheese made from goat or sheep's milk. Use them as a garnish over tender shellfish or a freshly cooked farm egg. Chives also make the perfect salad dressing booster for those who find garlic and raw onion to be too strong.

CILANTRO, a lemony, floral-flavored herb with lacy leaves, is prevalent in Mexican and Asian cooking. It imparts a bright flavor profile to fresh vegetables and is particularly well paired with white proteins such as chicken or fish. It can also lift the earthy taste of beans, potatoes, and mushrooms. If you are new to cilantro, try it cooked first, as it's mellower, and then graduate to raw. Cilantro works well in most recipes that call for basil and makes a tasty "South-of-the-Border" pesto when blended with garlic and olive oil.

MINT isn't just for garnishing desserts—it will bring a touch of sweetness wherever you add it, from veggie-based smoothies to soups and even to salads. Use it to make homemade teas sweeter without adding sugar. It pairs well with fruits such as berries and avocado, and vegetables such as zucchini and peas. It's a refreshing addition to cold preparations such as chilled seafood, gazpacho, and chicken or tuna salad. Just like basil, it comes in many varieties, from apple to lemon and even chocolate.

PARSLEY, a fresh herb that's easy to find year-round, has a note of astringent, grassy green flavor. Go for flat-leaf parsley (sometimes called Italian parsley), since it's far more flavorful and easier to chop. Like basil and cilantro, it can be used in soups, in sauces, and on meats, and is often considered the "catchall" herb that most people know and like.

ROSEMARY, part of the mint family, is a bolder herb like thyme and is typically added to seasoning salts and meat marinades. The top phytonutrients in rosmarinic acid and rosmanol are powerful antioxidants, with more antioxidant power than vitamin E. Rosemary is oftentimes used dried, but it contains more active phytonutrients when fresh. It pairs well with more flavorful meats such as beef, lamb, and buffalo, but it is also tasty with chicken and pork. It's a delightful addition to your summer grilling when chopped fresh and added to marinades for grilled summer veggies. Start with 1 to 2 tablespoons chopped.

SAGE, like thyme and rosemary, is a stronger herb that can be used for grilling or in marinades. Since it has a powerful scent and flavor, use one leaf to start in most recipes, or achieve a milder flavor by frying it in a few teaspoons of olive oil over medium heat. Sage is delicious with roasted butternut squash or potatoes. Fried sage leaves can be mixed with popcorn, crumbled over cheese for a special cheese platter, or used as a garnish over cooked shrimp or chicken. Varieties of sage range from purple to pineapple to Russian.

TARRAGON, related to the sunflower, is a licorice-flavored herb that is used often in traditional French cuisine. It pairs well with a host of ingredients, from fresh tomatoes and grapefruit to artichokes and asparagus. You can add a few leaves to almost any fresh vegetable dish that needs a hint of anise. Pair it with fresh citrus or citrus zest for a delicious fish or chicken marinade, or enjoy it as a component of pesto when mixed with basil or parsley.

THYME, part of the mint family, has a pungent flavor that perks up almost any dishes, including soups, stews, roasted meats, mashes, and baked fish. Thyme has a stronger taste than many herbs, so use smaller amounts (about 1 teaspoon fresh thyme leaves to start) and combine it with more mild herbs such as parsley. Traditionally, thyme is added to intensify the flavor in herb mixes, such as herbes de

Provence, and comes in several varieties, such as lemon, lime, and lavender.

Spices

CARDAMOM, a spice that resembles black pepper, has a minty flavor and can be located in your standard spice offerings in any grocery store. Cardamom, an important ingredient in Indian cuisines and used often in chai and curry, also works well in both savory and sweet dishes. It's delicious with chicken and seafood, and it brings a nice element to sweet desserts made with juicy fruits such as berries, mangoes, and figs.

BLACK PEPPER adds a taste of earthy heat to any meal. Freshly grinding your pepper in a pepper mill or coffee grinder is the best way to bring out its flavor (pre-ground pepper tends to lose its spark sitting on the shelf).

CHILI powders have a smoky, sometimes hot flavor that adds another layer of savoriness to your meal. They range from mild to hot, but either way you should look for chili powders that are salt- and sugar-free, made with ground chiles alone. If you are not a fan of spiciness, start with mild chili powder and gradually add a pinch of hotter ground chile, such as cayenne, to

build your tolerance to the heat. Chipotle chiles in adobo sauce are popular smoky, rich-tasting chiles that come canned in a spicy tomato sauce. Look for canned chipotle chiles in your local supermarket in the international aisle, or in a Latin American grocery store. Chile flakes, made up of chopped dried chiles and seeds, are a grocery store standard. They're perfect to perk up Italian fare, whether it be soups, cheese plates, or even antipasto. Add them to jarred marinara sauce for a zesty flavor boost.

CINNAMON, considered an American spice, is actually grown in India and Mexico. It is ideal for breakfast foods like hot cereals, French toast, and smoothies. Add a pinch of ground cinnamon to teas, coffees, and afternoon drinks to serve as fast, soothing aromatherapy. Sweet-tasting cinnamon can also be used in savory dishes, for example as part of a barbecue spice mix, brines, and roasts. Cinnamon pairs well with fruits, especially fall fruits such as apples and pears, and earthy nuts.

FENNEL SEEDS, often used in ground sausage, give off a sweet licorice perfume. Used as a natural breath freshener in India, fennel can also naturally sweeten spice mixes, while adding a nice contrast to spicy or hot ingredients like chiles. Fennel pairs well with pork, chicken, or beef.

GARLIC POWDER is a fast and flavorful way to bring in a garlicky taste, and it's a great option for people who don't digest raw garlic well. Garlic salt is just garlic powder with salt added in. If you're on a low-sodium diet, opt for garlic powder instead, and add your own salt according to your doctor's recommendations.

PUMPKIN PIE SPICE, a mix that usually contains a number of healing spices, including cinnamon, ginger, nutmeg, cloves, allspice, and white pepper, is used to flavor pumpkin pie. But don't banish it to the back of the spice rack—you can use it throughout the year for smoothies, soups, and breakfast cereals.

TURMERIC, considered nearly a panacea in both Eastern and Western medicine, is a powder ground from a dried rhizome that resembles ginger. It's easy to add this spice to dishes, from dressings to stews and soups and even desserts, but it does have a sour, pungent flavor that can overpower. It should be used in small quantities to start—try ¼ teaspoon for a recipe that serves four. Pair it with black pepper to increase the absorption of the active ingredient curcumin, one of the few molecules in food known to promote the expression of the brain growth factor, BDNF.

Cooking Fats

Think of the cooking fats in your kitchen as you do the oil in your car. You change the oil in your car every few months and you use only high-quality oil. The fats and oils in your diet should get the same attention. This is the place to avoid anything artificial. Please notice there are no weird, toxic fats from the laboratory like trans fats or interesterified fats in any of these recipes. Organic oils and fats are important to consider.

Here are a few fat guidelines.

- Don't eat fake fats.
- Use the lowest heat possible.
- Eat more MUFAs and PUFAs than saturated fats.
- Try to eat an equal balance of omega-3 and omega-6 fats. For most people, this means eating more seafood and eating less vegetable oil and meat.
- Use high-quality, organic fats and oil.
- Buy smaller bottles and store away from direct sunlight to prevent oxidation.
- Use them liberally with vegetables to improve nutrient absorption.

Only three fats are used in *Eat Complete*: olive oil, butter, and coconut oil.

OLIVE OIL. This fat is the most common fat in *Eat Complete.* Olive oil is unique as it is 75 percent oleic acid. This MUFA is the only fat all health experts seem to agree on! Olive oil contains a special phytonutrient, hydroxytryosol, known to protect the lining of your blood vessels and your brain's supply of oxygen. Use extra-virgin olive oil (EVOO), which contains more phytonutrients. Refined olive oils have higher smoke points and should be used for recipes that require higher heat.

GRASS-FED BUTTER. I recommend butter over margarine and whipped vegetable oils. This is based both on science and paranoia after the awful revelations about trans fats and other highly processed, industrial fats. Choosing grass-fed butter means more CLA, the fat that helps build muscle and seems to protect the heart. Certainly the best butter is spring butter; the deep yellow color means more carotenoids, the vitamin A precursors that create your sense of sight and that are key to brain development.

COCONUT OIL. Coconuts are unique in the plant world due to the high amounts of saturated fat. This fat works well for panfrying. A tablespoon in a smoothie adds creamy texture.

Essential Eat Complete Kitchen Tools

A BASIC SET OF TONGS that are easy to open and close will give you more control in cooking proteins and vegetables. They're dishwasher safe for easy cleanup and can be purchased for under five bucks.

PLASTIC CUTTING BOARDS are inexpensive and can be popped into your dishwasher so you don't have to hand wash them in between uses. Stock up on a few so that you can make prep faster and always have a clean one on hand. Solid wooden boards are my preference, though they must be replaced more often. Avoid wood cutting boards assembled with glue, which can contain formaldehyde.

A sharp **VEGETABLE PEELER** is a useful tool and is great for potato skins and even tougher peels such as mango skins. To protect the blades, wash this with soap and water rather than in the dishwasher. You can also put your kids to work in the kitchen by purchasing a child-safe peeler, like the Kyocera ceramic peeler for kids.

Grab a set of **INEXPENSIVE PARING KNIVES**, which are great for mincing garlic, slicing berries, and other general light food prep.

Zucchini noodles, carpaccio, and thin-sliced veggies are a snap when you use a **JAPANESE MANDOLIN** that's affordable and dishwasher safe. Alternatively, you can use a spiralizer to spiral your veggies into a healthier "noodle."

A MICROPLANE GRATER with sharp teeth will be your best friend when it comes to grating nutmeg, garlic cloves, and citrus zest. Slide it into your dishwasher for easy cleanup.

KITCHEN SHEARS come in handy when you want a quick herb garnish without getting out the cutting board. Shears are also great for cutting chicken breast into tenders or clipping away excess fats. Stainless steel blades make them dishwasher safe, and many versions come apart for even better cleanup.

A sturdy set of **BASIC KNIVES** is a must. I recommend an 8-inch chef's knife (depending on the size of your dominant hand), as well as a 10-inch serrated bread knife, and a good-quality paring knife (as discussed above). Hand washing your knives will allow them to last longer.

A MINI BLENDER is versatile and fits well in a small apartment kitchen. It is ideal for households of two, or serves as the perfect gift for a college freshman. The assortment of cups and the blade can be placed in the dishwasher for easy cleanup.

An **IMMERSION BLENDER** makes for easier cleanup and less mess by blending soups right in the stockpot. You can also make smoothies, pestos, or sauces with the push of a button. Many come with attachments that double as a mini chopper and electric whisk. The bottom detaches and can be popped right into the dishwasher.

For chopping, slicing, dicing, and shredding, a **FOOD PROCESSOR** will cut your prep time and is worthy of a prominent spot on your countertop. The food processor is great for batch cooking, such as making one of the many pestos, or to help you stock up on freezer meals (like the soups from this book).

With larger, more powerful motors, **BLENDERS** such as Vitamix and Blendtec won't stop until your smoothies, veggies, and sauces are silky smooth. While expensive, they will change how you make smoothies and soups, allowing you to add more nuts and veggies. Some lower-cost options exist. Get the sturdiest, highest-

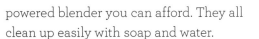
powered blender you can afford. They all clean up easily with soap and water.

Cook your grains and rice perfectly every time with a **RICE COOKER** that's smart enough to sense and adjust the heat. For anything from the amaranth breakfast cereal on page 129 to black rice on page 158, I rely on my Zojirushi rice cooker.

One large **STAINLESS STEEL SKILLET** and one small are all you'll need to make many of the recipes in this book. These tough skillets will last a lifetime.

NONSTICK SKILLETS with Teflon are a thing of the past (don't go down the rabbit hole of C8 and "Teflon flu"); instead, opt for something safer such as a cast-iron skillet that's easy to handle and clean. Cooking with cast iron is especially important for vegetarians as it increases the iron content.

If you plan to do any preserving or canning and want to regularly make stocks, a **LARGE STOCKPOT** will liberate you from the confines of your pasta pot.

Finally, a fermentation vessel such as a **LARGE STONEWARE CROCK** and a collection of glass jars make the brewing of pickles, sauerkrauts, kefir, kombucha, and sourdoughs much more satisfying. These tools help your kitchen come alive—literally.

Breakfast

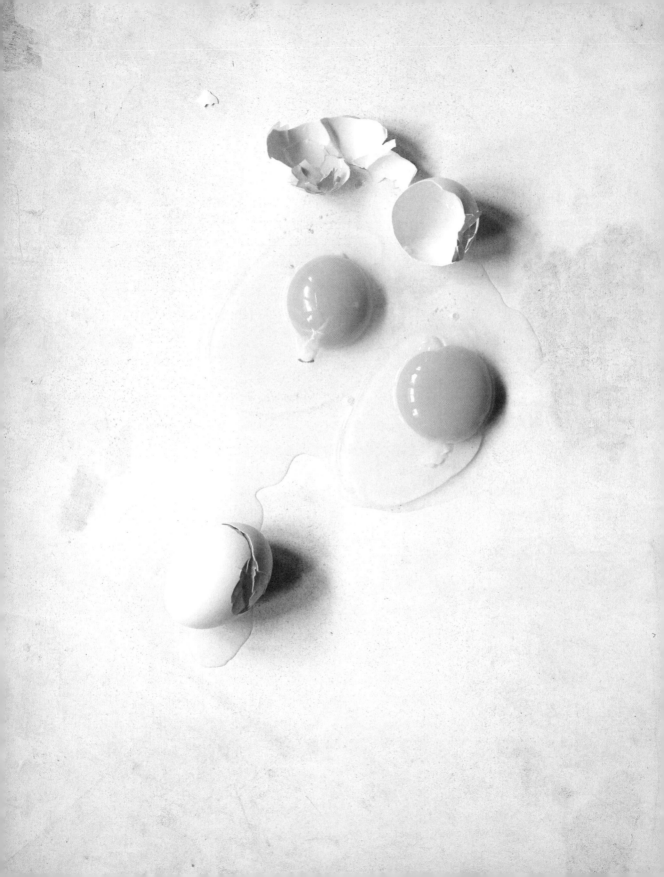

Kiwi Green Smoothie SERVES 2

You might be skeptical about starting your day with four cups of greens, but that will quickly pass. Mixing greens into your smoothies is an easy way to boost nutrient intake. The fiber in the greens plus the protein in the kefir will keep you full longer, and the live cultures in the yogurt or kefir promote overall gut health. To avoid bitterness, be sure your kiwis are ripe, which means they should be soft to the touch. Leave hard kiwis on the countertop for two to three days to ripen.

2 cups raw fresh spinach
2 cups raw kale
2 ripe kiwis, peeled and
    quartered

1 cup plain 2 percent yogurt
    or plain kefir
¼ cup almonds
¼ cup chia seeds

2 tablespoons honey
4 ice cubes
1 cup cold water, plus more
    as needed

Place the spinach, kale, kiwis, yogurt or kefir, almonds, chia seeds, and honey in a blender along with the ice cubes and cold water. Blend until smooth, adding a few tablespoons more of cold water to adjust the consistency if necessary. Divide evenly between two glasses and serve immediately.

NUTRITIONAL STATS PER SERVING (2 CUPS):
434 Calories ❖ 19g Protein ❖ 58g Carbohydrates ❖ 20g Fat (1g Saturated) ❖ 5mg Cholesterol ❖ 31g Sugars ❖ 19g Fiber ❖ 156mg Sodium

Vitamin K = 308% ❖ Vitamin C = 260% ❖ Fiber, Magnesium = 80% ❖ Vitamin A = 52% ❖ Protein = 43%

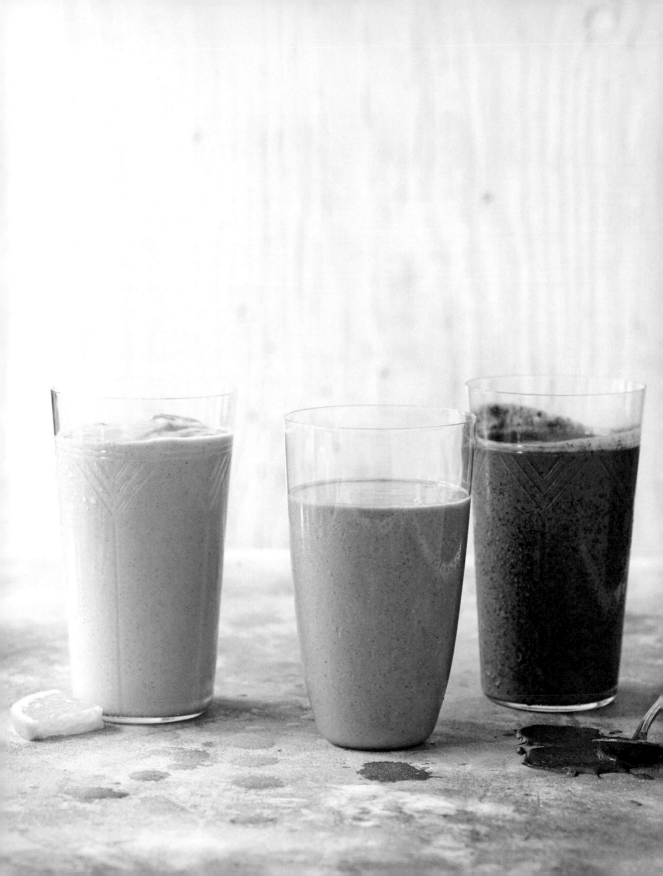

Minty Blueberry Shake SERVES 2

This is a breakfast that hits the mark for protein and taste, and it also happens to come with its own aromatherapy treatment. Mint calms and refreshes, so start your day by tearing up the mint leaves and taking a deep mindful breath. Pairing blueberries with greens gives you a powerful dose of plant-based medicine (see phytonutrients page 62), and covers your bases for your vitamin needs. The juicy wild blueberries plus an added subtle sweetness from the mint pair well with the vegetal taste of the greens.

2 cups fresh or frozen wild blueberries

1 cup plain, 2 percent yogurt or plain kefir

1 cup assorted greens such as spinach, baby kale, or collards

1 banana

¼ cup fresh mint leaves

¼ cup hemp seeds

¼ cup pumpkin seeds

4 ice cubes

¾ cup cold water

Place the blueberries, yogurt or kefir, greens, banana, mint leaves, hemp seeds, and pumpkin seeds in a blender along with the ice cubes and cold water and process until smooth. Divide evenly between two glasses and serve immediately.

Frozen berries are a great way to trim your grocery shopping budget while still preserving the nutrients. They also create a vibrant purple color and add a creamy texture to the shake.

NUTRITIONAL STATS PER SERVING (2 CUPS): 482 Calories ❖ 23g Protein ❖ 53g Carbohydrates ❖ 24g Fat (4g Saturated) ❖ 5mg Cholesterol ❖ 26g Sugars ❖ 11g Fiber ❖ 94mg Sodium

Vitamin C = 80% ❖ Magnesium = 75% ❖ Protein = 50% ❖ Fiber = 44% ❖ Iron = 28%

Cashew-Chocolate Smoothie SERVES 2

This is another phytonutrient fest! Start the day with two great sources of healthy monounsaturated fats: avocados and cashews. Nutrient-dense avocado thickens this smoothie beautifully while providing beneficial fats that boost brain health and enhance the beauty of your skin. Nuts such as cashews are a top source of plant-based antioxidants and essential minerals such as zinc, magnesium, and iron. The almond extract is an essential addition as it balances the avocado and cocoa.

1 cup plain, 2 percent yogurt or plain kefir

1 ripe Hass avocado

½ cup grass-fed whole milk

½ cup raw spinach

4 tablespoons chopped cashews

3 tablespoons unsweetened cocoa powder

3 tablespoons honey

¼ teaspoon pure almond extract

8 ice cubes

Place the yogurt or kefir, avocado, milk, spinach, half of the cashews, the cocoa powder, honey, and almond extract in a blender along with the ice cubes. Process until smooth, adding a few tablespoons of cold water to adjust the consistency if necessary. Divide evenly between two glasses, add 1 tablespoon of chopped cashews on top of each smoothie, and serve immediately.

NUTRITIONAL STATS PER SERVING (1½ CUPS):
364 Calories ❖ 11g Protein ❖ 47g Carbohydrates ❖ 18g Fat (4g Saturated) ❖ 11mg Cholesterol ❖ 33g Sugars ❖ 8g Fiber ❖ 103mg Sodium

Vitamin K = 67% ❖ Vitamin D = 41% ❖ Fiber = 32% ❖ Calcium = 25% ❖ Protein = 24%

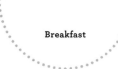
Buttermilk Strawberry Smoothie SERVES 2

Buttermilk, a cultured dairy product, adds zip to this berry delicious smoothie that's high in vitamin C and key minerals. Including cultured dairy in your diet benefits your health by adding good bacteria to your microbiome. If you can't do dairy, try cultured coconut yogurt instead.

1 cup 2 percent buttermilk
1 cup plain kefir
3 cups fresh strawberries

¼ cup almonds
2 tablespoons pumpkin seeds

1 teaspoon pure vanilla extract
8 ice cubes

Place the buttermilk, kefir, strawberries, almonds, pumpkin seeds, and vanilla in a blender along with the ice cubes. Process until smooth, adding a few tablespoons of cold water to adjust the consistency if necessary. Divide evenly between two glasses and serve immediately.

NUTRITIONAL STATS PER SERVING (2½ CUPS):
330 Calories ❖ 12g Protein ❖ 36g Carbohydrates ❖ 16g Fat (3g Saturated) ❖ 9mg Cholesterol ❖ 26g Sugars ❖ 6g Fiber ❖ 112mg Sodium

Vitamin C = 172% ❖ Magnesium = 45% ❖ Vitamin E = 30% ❖ Protein = 26% ❖ Fiber = 24%

Buttermilk comes in quarts in your local grocery and keeps in your fridge for up to 3 weeks. Look for buttermilk from grass-fed cows, or opt for one from a local farm. Enjoy the remaining buttermilk in the other tasty recipes in the book that call for it, such as Orange-Pecan Waffles (page 133), Artichoke-Leek Carpaccio with Buttermilk-Kefir Dressing (page 141), or Lentil and Mushroom Shepherd's Pie with Sweet Potato Topping (page 228).

Gingered Pumpkin Smoothie SERVES 2

Help preserve your brain with carotenoids, as these orange-yellow plant pigments come with a bevy of health benefits (and are linked to a decreased risk of dementia). This smoothie is based on creamy 100 percent organic canned pumpkin; pair that with a carrot, and you're starting the day with two top sources of beta-carotene. The recipe calls for only 1 cup of pumpkin, so preserve the remainder in the refrigerator in an airtight container, or freeze if you aren't planning to use it again within five days. The ginger makes the recipe pop. Add curry powder and black pepper and you're in for a savory nutritious treat; the pepper unlocks the benefits of curry by increasing its absorption by 2,000 percent.

- 1 cup 100 percent pure organic canned pumpkin
- 1 orange, peeled
- 1 carrot, peeled and chopped
- ½ cup plain, 2 percent yogurt or plain kefir
- ¼ cup sunflower seeds
- ¼ cup cashews
- 1 tablespoon peeled and grated fresh ginger
- ½ teaspoon pure vanilla extract
- 1 teaspoon pumpkin pie spice
- 1 teaspoon curry powder (optional)
- Dash of freshly ground black pepper
- 4 ice cubes
- ½ cup cold water

Place the pumpkin, orange, carrot, yogurt or plain kefir, sunflower seeds, cashews, ginger, vanilla, pumpkin pie spice, curry powder, if using, and pepper in a blender along with the ice cubes and cold water and process until smooth. Divide evenly between two glasses and serve immediately.

Turmeric (an ingredient in curry powder) is a superspice in the ginger family that has wide-reaching healing benefits due to its anti-inflammatory properties. This yellow spice makes for a nice addition to this smoothie without altering its fruity flavor. Shop for turmeric in the spice aisle of your local grocery store.

NUTRITIONAL STATS PER SERVING (2 CUPS):
328 Calories ❖ 11g Protein ❖ 35g Carbohydrates ❖ 19g Fat (3g Saturated) ❖ 2.5mg Cholesterol ❖ 14g Sugars ❖ 10g Fiber ❖ 63mg Sodium

Vitamin A = 179% ❖ Vitamin C = 57% ❖ Fiber = 40% ❖ Vitamin K = 36% ❖ Magnesium = 35%

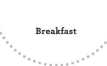
Balsamic Strawberry Parfait SERVES 4

Balsamic vinegar may seem a strange addition to this otherwise classic parfait, but balsamic drizzled over strawberries is a classic Italian combo that makes for a sweet and sour taste sensation. Want to take these on the road with you? They are perfect for a summer picnic dessert when assembled in mason jars.

½ cup almonds, chopped
¼ cup chia seeds
2 tablespoons brown sugar

¼ teaspoon ground cinnamon
3 tablespoons water
2 tablespoons balsamic vinegar

2 cups strawberries, hulled and diced
½ cup cooked quinoa
4 cups plain whole milk Greek yogurt

Put the almonds in a small saucepan over medium-low heat and toast for 2 to 3 minutes, stirring occasionally, until the almonds start to brown. Add the chia seeds, brown sugar, and cinnamon along with the water. Increase the heat to medium and cook for about 1 minute more until the mixture starts to bubble. Turn the heat off and add the vinegar, strawberries, and quinoa and stir well.

Set out four parfait glasses and, using a spatula, add ½ cup of the yogurt to each glass. Top with a few tablespoons of the strawberry-nut mixture, then another ½ cup of yogurt. Top with the remaining strawberry-nut mixture and serve immediately, or cover with plastic wrap and refrigerate. Consume within 2 days.

NUTRITIONAL STATS PER SERVING (1½ CUPS):
376 Calories ❖ 25g Protein ❖ 34g Carbohydrates ❖ 19g Fat (3g Saturated) ❖ 13mg Cholesterol ❖ 18g Sugars ❖ 10g Fiber ❖ 65mg Sodium

Vitamin C and Protein = 56% ❖ Fiber = 40% ❖ Magnesium = 38% ❖ Calcium = 28% ❖ Iodine = 23%

Quinoa-Mushroom Frittata with Fresh Herbs SERVES 6

Used as healing compounds since the early days of medicine, herbs have strong scents and flavors that indicate the presence of unique phytonutrients. Study after study shows that traditional healers were right: these plants are medicine. This simple dish brings some serious plant power with the fresh herbs, mushrooms, olives, and quinoa. Mushrooms also contain unique phytonutrients, helping you round out this meal. For your next brunch, serve up some healing!

¾ cup uncooked quinoa (or 1½ cups cooked)

6 large pasture-raised eggs

½ cup grated Parmesan cheese

¼ cup chopped fresh basil

2 tablespoons chopped fresh chives or tarragon

1 teaspoon minced fresh thyme leaves

¼ teaspoon freshly ground black pepper

4 green onions or garlic scapes, thinly sliced

1 cup sliced mushrooms such as maitake, shiitake, or chanterelle, brushed clean and sliced

Olive oil

¼ cup assorted pitted olives, whole or chopped

Cook the quinoa according to the package instructions. Set aside.

In a large bowl, whisk the eggs, then stir in the quinoa, Parmesan, herbs, pepper, green onions or garlic scapes, and mushrooms.

Coat a medium, ovenproof skillet with a thick layer of olive oil. Place over medium-high heat, add the egg mixture, and sprinkle with the olives. Cook for 2 to 3 minutes without stirring.

Preheat the broiler with the rack in the second position from the top. Broil the frittata until the top is lightly browned and the eggs have firmed up in the center, 3 to 4 minutes.

Remove the frittata from the oven and let it rest for 3 minutes. Loosen the edges with a spatula and cut into 6 wedges. Serve immediately.

NUTRITIONAL STATS PER SERVING (1 LARGE WEDGE): 232 Calories ❖ 13g Protein ❖ 14g Carbohydrates ❖ 14g Fat (6g Saturated) ❖ 295mg Cholesterol ❖ 2g Sugars ❖ 2g Fiber ❖ 409mg Sodium

Selenium = 65% ❖ Vitamin K = 51% ❖ B_{12} = 39% ❖ Choline = 35% ❖ Zinc = 33%

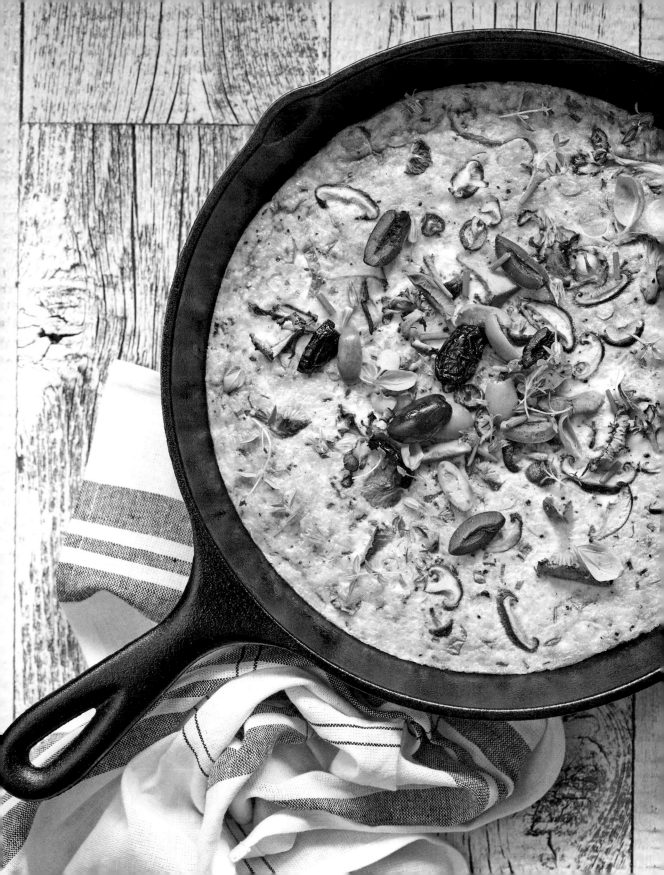

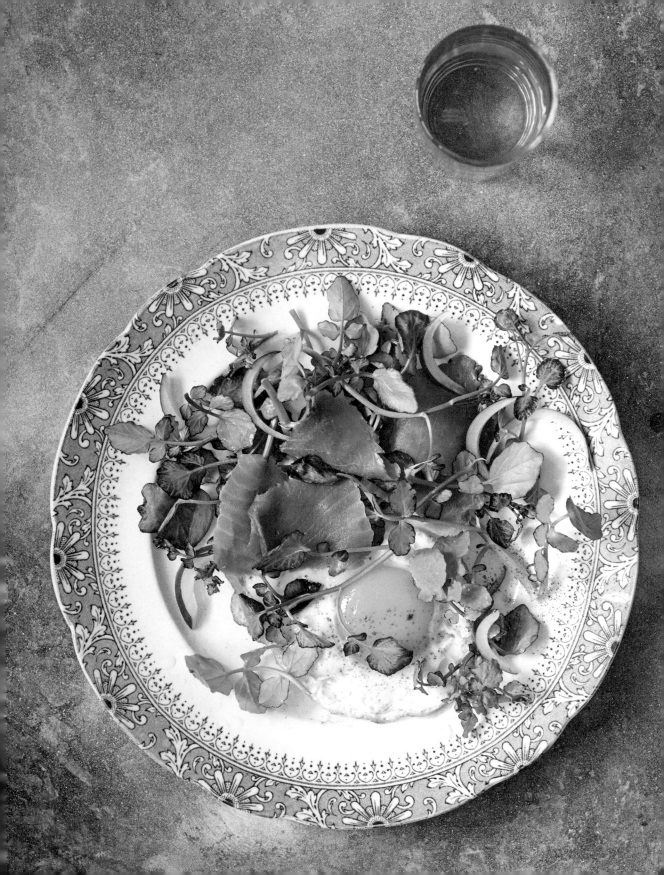

Truffled Farm Egg with Wilted Watercress and Smoked Salmon SERVES 4

As a trio, seafood, greens, and eggs in this dish deliver all of the essential 21 nutrients. For even more omega-3s (and no food dyes), choose wild salmon, which is sometimes harder to find than smoked salmon. Another option is to make your own cured salmon, using the homemade gravlax recipe on page 183. Watercress tops the rankings of fruits and vegetables for overall nutrient density. To take this brunch-style breakfast on the go, wrap your eggs and fixings in a large collard leaf, which boosts the nutrient density of the dish. Serious foodies can swap the truffle oil for 2 teaspoons shaved fresh truffle, black or white, added to 2 teaspoons olive oil.

1 tablespoon olive oil
4 pasture-raised eggs
2 teaspoons truffle oil

1 teaspoon paprika
1 shallot or ½ red onion,
 thinly sliced
8 ounces watercress

2 tablespoons balsamic or
 apple cider vinegar
8 ounces smoked salmon

Coat a large skillet with half of the olive oil and warm it over medium-high heat. Crack the eggs into the skillet, drizzle with the truffle oil, and sprinkle with paprika. Cook for 3 to 4 minutes until the whites are cooked through but the yolks are still soft.

While the eggs are cooking, prepare the watercress. Coat a separate large skillet with the remaining olive oil. Add the shallot or onion and cook for 2 to 3 minutes until the shallot starts to soften. Add the watercress and cook for 1 minute until wilted. Sprinkle with the vinegar.

Divide the mixture among four plates and top each with an egg and 2 ounces of the smoked salmon. Serve immediately.

NUTRITIONAL STATS PER SERVING: 387 Calories 30g Protein ❖ 4g Carbohydrates ❖ 27g Fat (6g Saturated) ❖ 246mg Cholesterol ❖ 3g Sugars ❖ .5g Fiber ❖ 489mg Sodium

Vitamin K = 160% ❖ EPA+DHA = 60% ❖ Choline = 45% ❖ Vitamin C = 33% ❖ Selenium and Iodine = 29%

Avocado Baked Egg with Roasted Red Pepper Coulis SERVES 4

Chock-full of choline and B vitamins, eggs and avocados are two nutrient-rich foods that have been unfairly spurned in the era of low-fat foods. Both offer a nice mix of fats, protein, and phytonutrients, and they even come in their own biodegradable containers. Egg yolks have a bad reputation, but I recommend eating them as they contain most of an egg's nutrients—including choline, a lack of which is linked to higher anxiety levels. With this dish, there is no need to worry about what's for breakfast. And as a bonus, leftover coulis makes a mean salad dressing—you can adjust the consistency with a few teaspoons of cold water.

3 red bell peppers
4 Hass avocados
8 pasture-raised eggs

1 shallot, peeled and chopped
1 tablespoon olive oil
1 tablespoon sherry vinegar or red wine vinegar

¼ teaspoon salt
⅛ teaspoon freshly ground black pepper

Cover a baking sheet with aluminum foil. Place the bell peppers on the baking sheet and place under the broiler. Broil 3 to 4 minutes, turning often, until the skins are charred. Transfer to a bowl, cover, and let steam.

Preheat the oven to 425°F. Slice the avocados in half, and remove and discard the pits. Scoop out 1 tablespoon of flesh from the center of each avocado to allow the egg to fit snugly in the center. Reserve avocado.

Place the avocados in a small 8 × 8-inch baking dish, so they fit tightly and don't tip over. Crack an egg into each avocado half. Bake in the oven for 15 to 20 minutes until the whites have set and are cooked through.

While the egg is baking, prepare the coulis. Peel the blackened skin from the peppers and discard. Remove the seeds and discard. Chop the peppers and transfer to a blender along with the shallot, olive oil, vinegar, salt, and black pepper. Blend until smooth. When the avocado eggs have finished cooking, garnish each plate with reserved fresh avocado, drizzle with the coulis, and serve immediately.

NUTRITIONAL STATS PER SERVING (1 BAKED AVOCADO WITH COULIS): 249 Calories ❖ 9g Protein ❖ 14g Carbohydrates ❖ 18g Fat (4g Saturated) ❖ 186mg Cholesterol ❖ 4g Sugars ❖ 8g Fiber ❖ 221mg Sodium

Vitamin C = 136% ❖ Choline = 69% ❖ Iodine = 36% ❖ Fiber = 33% ❖ Selenium, Vitamin A = 28%

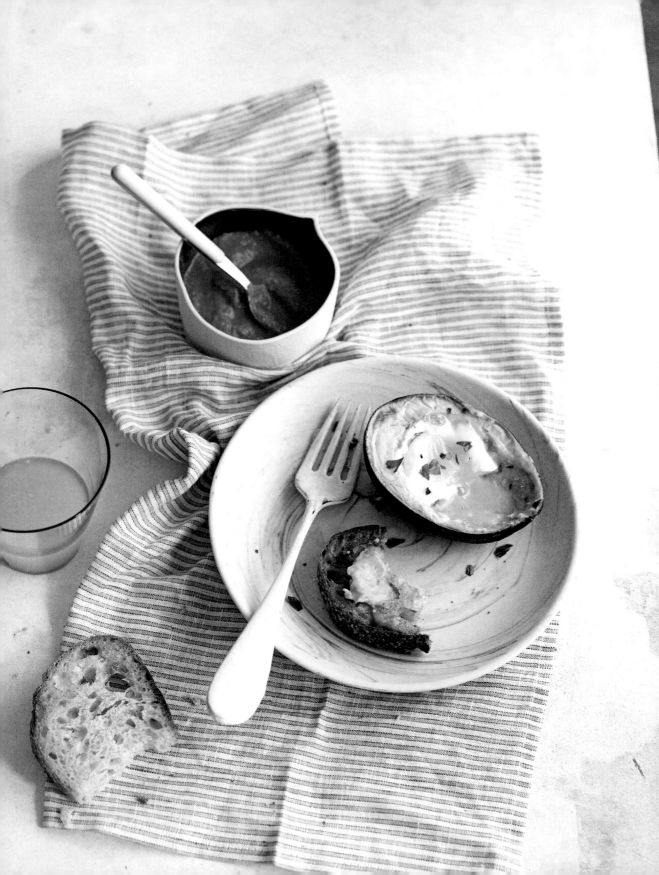

Baked Eggs in Crispy Kale Cups SERVES 4

This recipe upgrades your average plate of bacon and eggs into a more nutritious start to your day. The carotenoids in the kale help preserve your vision, and eggs are a top source of choline and B vitamins, and carotenoids instead of cholesterol. In the brain, choline is responsible for making acetylcholine, a workhouse molecule involved in learning. This quick, easy breakfast yields crispy cruciferous leaves that are perfect for dipping in the soft egg yolk. To make this dish heartier, top each egg with ½ teaspoon pesto (page 214) before baking.

Olive oil
8 large kale leaves, cut in half
4 pasture-raised eggs
4 slices prosciutto

Preheat the oven to 400°F. Grease a 12-cup muffin pan with a light coating of olive oil. Press 4 of the kale leaves into 4 of the cups and crack an egg into each one. Place the remaining kale into 4 other cups. Press a prosciutto slice into the last 4 cups.

Bake for 10 to 15 minutes until the whites of the eggs are cooked through and the kale and prosciutto are crisp. Place an egg on each plate and divide the remaining kale and prosciutto equally among the four plates

NUTRITIONAL STATS PER SERVING (ONE EGG PLUS PROSCIUTTO AND EXTRA KALE): 156
Calories ❖ 12g Protein ❖ 5g Carbohydrates ❖ 10g Fat (2.5g Saturated) ❖ 193mg Cholesterol ❖ 1g Sugars ❖ 1g Fiber ❖ 467mg Sodium

Vitamin K = 610% ❖ Vitamin C = 107% ❖ Vitamin A = 85% ❖ Choline = 35% ❖ Selenium = 29%

Homemade Kefir Served with Hot Cinnamon-Apple Slices SERVES 4

Kefir is a fermented milk drink made with kefir "grains," which are a form of SCOBY (Symbiotic Colony of Bacteria and Yeast) used as a starter. Fermenting your own kefir is simple, and rewarding, with delicious results. The starter "grains" contain a mixture of billions of health-promoting bacteria such as *Lactobacillus* and *Bifidobacter*, which consume the lactose in the milk. Vegans or other dairy-free folks can instead ferment coconut milk or another dairy-free milk. If making kefir seems daunting, shop for plain, unflavored kefir to use as a base for this recipe and others in the book. Skip the flavored kefirs, as these come with a lot of added sugar.

1 tablespoon kefir grains

1 quart grass-fed 2 percent milk

1 tablespoon olive oil

2 apples, thinly sliced

2 tablespoons brown sugar

½ teaspoon ground cinnamon

2 tablespoons water

Place the kefir grains and the milk in a glass jar and cover tightly. Set out at room temperature for 12 to 14 hours. Shake the jar gently a few times throughout the fermenting period. When your kefir is ready, you will see kefir grains coagulate on the top. Strain the grains to use in the next batch.

Store the kefir, refrigerated, for 3 to 4 weeks.

For the apple topping, warm the olive oil in a large skillet over medium heat. Add the apples and cook for 3 to 4 minutes, turning occasionally, until the apples have begun to soften. Reduce the heat to low and add the brown sugar and cinnamon along with the water. Toss well and cook for 2 minutes more until the apples are soft. Place ½ cup of the kefir in each of four bowls and divide the apples among the bowls. Reserve the remaining kefir for another use.

NUTRITIONAL STATS PER SERVING (1 CUP OF KEFIR AND APPLES): 173 Calories ❖ 6g Protein ❖ 20g Carbohydrates ❖ 6g Fat (2g Saturated) ❖ 10mg Cholesterol ❖ 22g Sugars ❖ 2g Fiber ❖ 78mg Sodium

Iodine = 37% ❖ Vitamin D = 26% ❖ B_{12} = 22% ❖ Calcium = 20% ❖ Protein = 13%

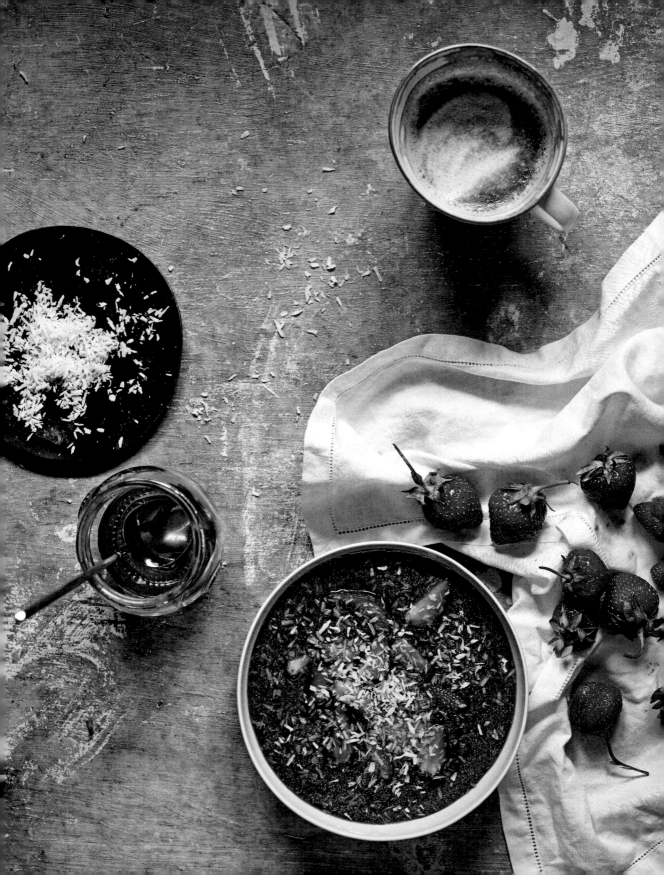

Chocolate Hot Amaranth Breakfast Cereal SERVES 4

Worried that your sweet tooth and love of chocolate will get in the way of eating complete? Think again. Ancient grains such as amaranth are a simple way to boost your nutrient intake, and they can be easily flavored with cocoa powder and honey. A staple food of the Aztecs, amaranth is a tiny grain, high in the minerals magnesium and manganese, which cooks in less than 30 minutes. Look for amaranth in your local health food store, or shop in bulk online and store bags in your freezer or fridge to extend their shelf life.

1½ cups amaranth
3½ cups water

2 tablespoons unsweetened cocoa powder
1 tablespoon honey

¼ cup unsweetened shredded coconut
2 cups diced strawberries

Place the amaranth in a large saucepan along with the water and bring to a boil over medium heat. Reduce the heat to a simmer and cook, stirring every 5 to 8 minutes, until creamy, 20 to 25 minutes in total. During the last few minutes, stir in the cocoa powder. Turn off the heat and stir in the honey. If the porridge seems too thick, add a few tablespoons of water. Sprinkle with coconut and berries and serve.

NUTRITIONAL STATS PER SERVING (1½ CUPS):
356 Calories ❖ 10g Protein ❖ 62g Carbohydrates ❖ 8g Fat (3g Saturated) ❖ 0mg Cholesterol ❖ 10g Sugars ❖ 7g Fiber ❖ 32mg Sodium

Magnesium = 49% ❖ Zinc = 29% ❖ Fiber = 28% ❖ Protein = 22% ❖ Iron = 14%

Sourdough Blueberry Pancakes with Kiwi–Red Currant Sauce SERVES 4

This simple sourdough pancake uses fermentation to create lofty, complex flavors and unlock the rich nutrition in grains. Instead of a sugar bomb, these pancakes give you a more complex brew of minerals, vitamins, and fats. This recipe is also great using a live sourdough starter. (For more information on sourdough starters, see page 33.)

Pancakes
- 1 10-gram packet sourdough starter
- 1 cup grass-fed whole milk
- 1 cup gluten-free or whole-grain pancake mix
- 1 cup finely chopped walnuts
- 1 cup fresh or frozen blueberries
- 1 pasture-raised egg
- 2 tablespoons olive oil or grass-fed butter

Sauce
- 1 cup red currants, stems removed
- ¼ cup water
- 1 tablespoon honey
- 2 kiwis, peeled and diced

Prepare the pancake batter the night before. In a medium glass bowl, soak 1 teaspoon of the dried starter in 1 tablespoon warm water for 10 minutes. Stir in the milk and the pancake mix. Cover with a clean towel. Rest on the countertop overnight; the mixture will bubble a bit.

The next morning, add the nuts, berries, egg, and 1 tablespoon oil or butter. Stir until a loose batter forms and set aside.

Prepare the sauce: Place the currants in a saucepan with the water. Add the honey and bring to a simmer over medium-low heat. Cook for 2 to 3 minutes until the currants soften and the mixture thickens. Cool for 5 minutes, then stir in half the kiwi.

Coat a griddle or cast-iron skillet with the remaining oil or butter. Place over medium-high heat. Drop the batter by scant ¼ cups onto the griddle or skillet, 1 inch apart. Cook for 2 to 3 minutes until the edges start to brown. Flip and cook for 2 to 3 minutes more. Repeat making pancakes with the remaining batter.

Set out 4 plates and place 3 pancakes onto each plate, then cover with fruit sauce and the remaining kiwi. Serve immediately.

NUTRITIONAL STATS PER SERVING (THREE 3-INCH PANCAKES WITH ⅓ CUP SAUCE): 444
Calories ❖ 10g Protein ❖ 56g Carbohydrates ❖ 22g Fat (3g Saturated) ❖ 51mg Cholesterol ❖ 14g Sugars ❖ 4g Fiber ❖ 329mg Sodium

ALA = 304% ❖ Protein = 23% ❖ Calcium, Magnesium = 20% ❖ Thiamine, Zinc = 18% ❖ Fiber = 16%

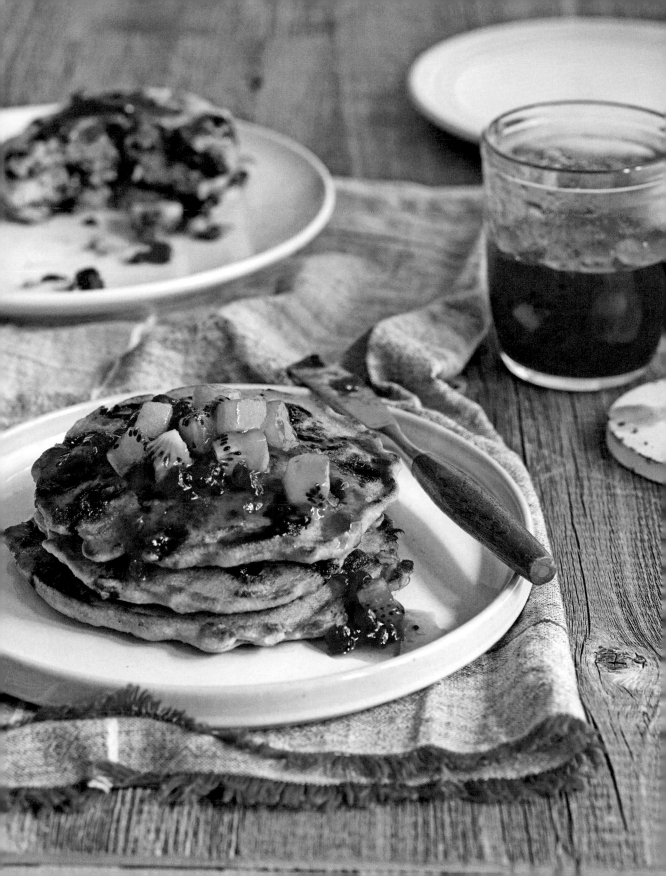

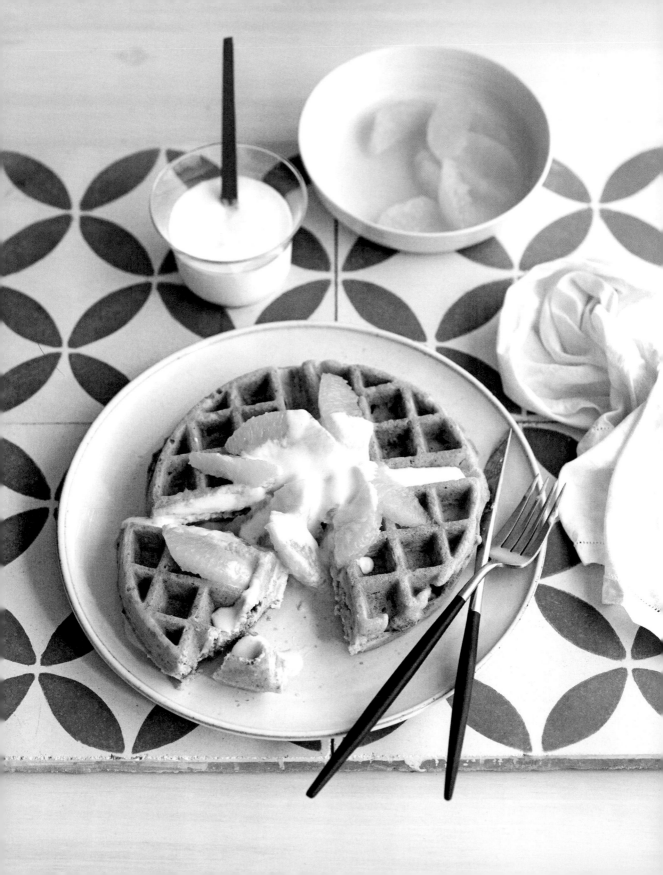

Orange-Pecan Waffles SERVES 4

Add nuts, seeds, and zest to your waffles to deliver fiber, flavor, and phytonutrients. Pecans are rich in vitamin E, an important protector of brain fat, and the zest of the citrus stimulates your opioid receptors, a key regulator of pleasure. High in fiber, low in sugar, these waffles ensure that you start the day with protein, calcium, and magnesium and help you ditch sugary OJ for an orange. It's time to get your waffle iron out. Use your sourdough starter for a fermented variation.

- 1 cup gluten-free pancake mix
- 1 cup cooked amaranth, millet, or quinoa
- ½ cup chopped pecans
- ½ cup buttermilk or whole milk, preferably from grass-fed cows
- 1 pasture-raised egg
- 2 tablespoons chia seeds
- 2 oranges, zested
- 3 tablespoons cold water
- Olive oil
- 1 cup plain kefir

Combine the pancake mix; amaranth, millet, or quinoa; and the pecans, milk, egg, chia seeds, and orange zest in a large bowl. Add the cold water and stir until a loose batter forms. Set aside to rest for 5 minutes to allow the chia seeds to thicken the mixture slightly.

Meanwhile, prepare the oranges. Remove the pith and the remaining peel with a small sharp knife. Working over a small bowl to catch the juices, remove the orange segments, discarding the membrane, and place the segments in the bowl with the juices.

Coat a waffle iron with olive oil. Preheat the waffle iron according to the manufacturer's instructions. Pour ½ cup of the batter into the waffle iron and close the lid. Cook until the indicator light signals that the waffle is cooked through. Transfer to a plate and repeat making waffles with the remaining batter.

Top each waffle with one-quarter of the orange segments and ¼ cup of the kefir. Serve immediately. To save time, make waffles in batches and store. To freeze, allow the waffles to cool completely and transfer to zipper-lock bags. Freeze for up to 6 months, or refrigerate for up to 1 week.

NUTRITIONAL STATS PER SERVING (1 WAFFLE WITH ¼ CUP TOPPING): 444 Calories ❖ 12g Protein ❖ 65g Carbohydrates ❖ 17g Fat (3g Saturated) ❖ 57mg Cholesterol ❖ 12g Sugars ❖ 8g Fiber ❖ 355mg Sodium

Vitamin C = 47% ❖ Fiber = 32% ❖ Magnesium = 29% ❖ Calcium = 28% ❖ Protein = 27%

Cacao Nib–Pepita Granola   MAKES 5 CUPS GRANOLA

Cacao nibs are energizing and increase blood flow to the brain. In clinical trials, dark chocolate has been shown to improve mood, focus, and memory. When you need a pick-me-up to help you climb and conquer that mountain of work, choose chocolate, straight up, in cracked bean or cacao nib form. This granola combines the whole-grain goodness of oats with nutrient-dense chia and hemp seeds to make the perfect vehicle for a cacao nib snack. Remember to use gluten-free oats if you are cooking for people with celiac disease.

Olive oil
2 cups rolled oats
⅓ cup chia seeds
⅓ cup hemp seeds
½ cup shredded
   unsweetened coconut

¼ cup pumpkin seeds
   (*pepitas*)
2 tablespoons brown sugar
½ teaspoon ground
   cinnamon
¼ teaspoon salt

1 pasture-raised egg
2 tablespoons cold water
3 tablespoons cacao nibs
2 cups plain kefir

Preheat the oven to 300°F. Lightly grease two baking sheets with olive oil. In a large bowl, combine the oats, chia seeds, hemp seeds, coconut, pumpkin seeds, brown sugar, cinnamon, salt, and egg. Add the cold water and stir well. Divide the mixture between the two prepared baking sheets, spreading it out well.

Bake for 25 to 30 minutes, stirring every 15 minutes, until the oats and coconut begin to brown. Remove from the oven and transfer to a large bowl. Add the cacao nibs and mix until evenly distributed. Cool the granola completely before serving. Serve each portion with ½ cup of kefir.

NUTRITIONAL STATS PER SERVING (1 CUP): 379
Calories ❖ 14g Protein ❖ 36g Carbohydrates ❖ 23g Fat (6g Saturated) ❖ 37mg Cholesterol ❖ 5g Sugars ❖ 12g Fiber ❖ 134mg Sodium

Fiber = 48% ❖ Vitamin E = 40% ❖ Zinc = 34% ❖ Protein = 31% ❖ Iron = 23%

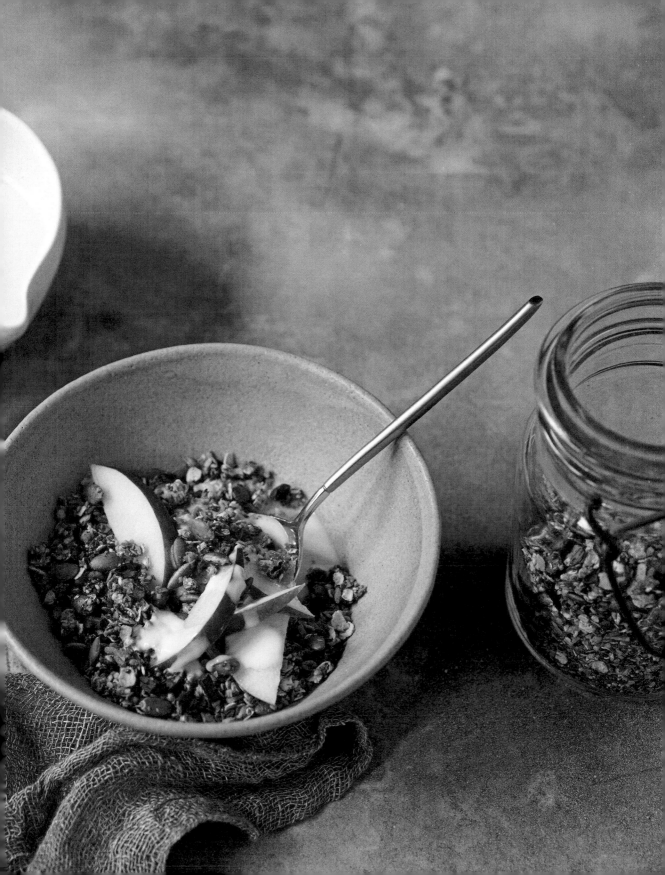

Spiced Carrot Bars MAKES 12 BARS

Carrot cake fans will cheer for this bar—it has the same flavorful profile, but with less sugar and more nutrients thanks to the carrots, pumpkin seeds, and chia seeds. Turn these tasty bars into a tempting dessert by adding a half cup of bittersweet chocolate morsels to the mix.

Olive oil cooking spray
4 carrots, peeled and grated
1 cup rolled oats
1 cup unsweetened shredded coconut

½ cup almond butter or peanut butter
½ cup raisins or dried cherries
⅓ cup chopped pumpkin seeds
¼ cup honey

2 pasture-raised eggs
2 tablespoons chia or hemp seeds
1 teaspoon baking soda
1 teaspoon pumpkin pie spice or ground cinnamon

Preheat the oven to 350°F. Spray a 9 × 11-inch baking pan with cooking spray.

In a large bowl, combine the carrots, oats, coconut, nut butter, raisins or cherries, pumpkin seeds, honey, eggs, chia or hemp seeds, baking soda, and pumpkin pie spice or cinnamon and stir well with a wooden spoon to form a stiff dough. Firmly press the dough into the prepared pan, using the back of a spoon. Bake for 25 to 30 minutes, or until the top is lightly browned. Cool in the pan on a rack.

To serve, cut into 12 squares. Store leftovers in an airtight container.

NUTRITIONAL STATS PER SERVING (1 BAR): 222
Calories ❖ 6g Protein ❖ 26g Carbohydrates ❖ 12g Fat (3g Saturated) ❖ 31mg Cholesterol ❖ 13g Sugars ❖ 4g Fiber ❖ 135mg Sodium

Vitamin A = 26% ❖ Magnesium = 22% ❖ Fiber = 16% ❖ Zinc = 15% ❖ Protein = 14%

Small Plates

Millet-Cheddar Fritters over Farm-Fresh Spinach SERVES 4

If you're a fan of scallion pancakes, you'll adore these gluten-free fritters that will also remind you of corn cakes. Millet has more protein and iron than many grains, along with high concentrations of polyphenol phytonutrients. To turn this into a main meal, double the recipe or make this whole recipe for two. For leftover fritters, cool completely and store in zipper-lock bags for a school or post-gym snack.

½ pound spinach or mustard greens, trimmed and chopped
1 tablespoon olive oil
1 cup cooked millet

1 cup grated cheddar cheese
4 scallions, thinly sliced
2 pasture-raised eggs
½ teaspoon paprika
½ teaspoon baking powder

¼ teaspoon freshly ground black pepper
¼ teaspoon garlic salt
Olive oil cooking spray
4 tablespoons jarred salsa

Toss the spinach or mustard greens in a large bowl with the olive oil. Arrange the spinach or mustard greens on four plates, dividing them equally.

Combine the millet in a bowl with the cheese, scallions, eggs, paprika, baking powder, pepper, and garlic salt. Stir until a thick mixture forms.

Coat a large ceramic or cast-iron skillet with olive oil cooking spray and place over medium-high heat. Drop the batter into the skillet (about 3 tablespoons per mound) and press the mounds down with a fork. Cook for 3 to 4 minutes until the cakes start to brown and the edges look translucent. Mist the top of the cakes with the cooking spray before turning. Flip and cook for 2 to 3 minutes more on the opposite sides until no longer wet in the center.

Place two cakes on each plate atop the greens, add 1 tablespoon salsa to each, and serve immediately.

NUTRITIONAL STATS PER SERVING (2 CAKES, SALSA, AND 1½ CUPS GREENS): 274 Calories ❖ 14g Protein ❖ 18g Carbohydrates ❖ 15g Fat (7g Saturated) ❖ 122mg Cholesterol ❖ 1g Sugars ❖ 2g Fiber ❖ 538mg Sodium

Vitamin K = 341% ❖ Vitamin A = 57% ❖ Folate = 36% ❖ Calcium = 33% ❖ Protein = 30%

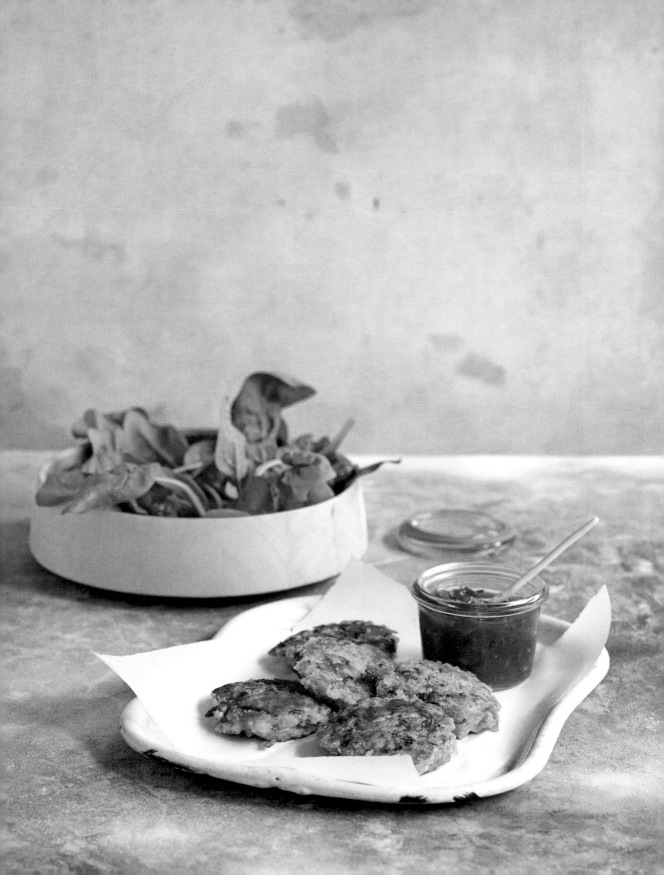

Kale-Artichoke Fritto Misto with Prebiotic Vinegar Dipping Sauce SERVES 4

Even the most vegetable-averse eater can be wooed by these crispy panfried vegetables. Raw apple cider vinegar is a prebiotic food that supports the health-promoting organisms in your gut and improves your digestion of simple sugars. Vinegar contains acetic acid, a short-chained fatty acid that is the preferred food of good gut bacteria. It also serves as the perfect dipping sauce for crispy panfried vegetables, which provide the other preferred food of a healthy microbiome: plant fibers. Look for raw apple cider vinegar in health food stores or in gourmet markets, and store it in a cool, dark place to protect its taste and color.

Dipping Sauce

6 tablespoons raw apple cider vinegar

2 tablespoons peeled and minced fresh ginger

1 tablespoon honey

Fritto Misto

¼ cup gluten-free pancake batter

2 ice cubes

2 tablespoons cold water

6 tablespoons olive oil

4 large kale leaves, quartered

8 frozen artichoke hearts, defrosted

8 shiitake mushrooms, stems removed and discarded

¼ teaspoon salt

Prepare the dipping sauce: Place the vinegar, ginger, and honey in a small bowl and stir well. Set the dipping sauce aside.

Make the fritto misto: Place the pancake batter in a large bowl along with the ice cubes and cold water, stir well, and set aside.

Line a baking sheet with paper towels. Heat the olive oil in a small heavy-bottomed saucepan over medium-high heat for about 1 minute. Just prior to coating the veggies, stir the pancake batter once again.

Working in batches, dip the veggies into the batter and then shake them free of excess batter. Place each piece in the oil

and panfry for about 1 minute, or until well browned. Remove with tongs and transfer to the prepared baking sheet. Sprinkle with a pinch of the salt while still hot. Repeat with the remaining vegetables and salt. Serve immediately with the dipping sauce.

NUTRITIONAL STATS PER SERVING (5 PIECES PLUS SAUCE): 273 Calories ❖ 3g Protein ❖ 21g Carbohydrates ❖ 21g Fat (2g Saturated) ❖ 0mg Cholesterol ❖ 5g Sugars ❖ 3g Fiber ❖ 259mg Sodium

Vitamin C = 60% ❖ Magnesium = 12% ❖ Vitamin A, Iron = 7% ❖ Potassium, Zinc = 6% ❖ Selenium, Thiamine = 5%

Artichoke-Leek Carpaccio with Buttermilk-Kefir Dressing SERVES 4

Carpaccio, a traditional Italian dish of thinly sliced tender meats or vegetables, is always enjoyed raw. Paper-thin slices are key, so search out a Japanese mandolin, an inexpensive slicing tool that gets the job done—no knife skills required. Your efforts will be rewarded with ample amounts of folate and magnesium, which help you relax and smile.

2 ounces pancetta, chopped

3 tablespoons red wine vinegar

2 tablespoons olive oil

½ teaspoon garlic salt

½ teaspoon Dijon mustard

2 anchovies, mashed

¼ teaspoon freshly ground black pepper

8 raw or frozen artichoke hearts, defrosted, thinly sliced

4 leeks, washed well and thinly sliced

Put the pancetta in a small cold skillet and place over medium heat. Cook for 4 to 5 minutes, stirring occasionally, until crispy. Transfer to a paper towel to drain and set aside. Reserve the fat in the skillet.

Place the skillet with the fat over low heat and add the vinegar, olive oil, garlic salt, mustard, anchovies, and pepper. Heat for 2 minutes and mix vigorously.

Spread out the artichokes and leeks on a large platter. Drizzle the warm dressing over the artichokes and leeks. Sprinkle with the pancetta and serve immediately.

NUTRITIONAL STATS PER SERVING (1½ CUPS):
291 Calories ❖ 11g Protein ❖ 41g Carbohydrates ❖ 12g Fat (3g Saturated) ❖ 6mg Cholesterol ❖ 6g Sugars ❖ 23g Fiber ❖ 527mg Sodium

Vitamin K = 91% ❖ Fiber = 92% ❖ Folate = 68% ❖ Magnesium = 40% ❖ Vitamin C = 38%

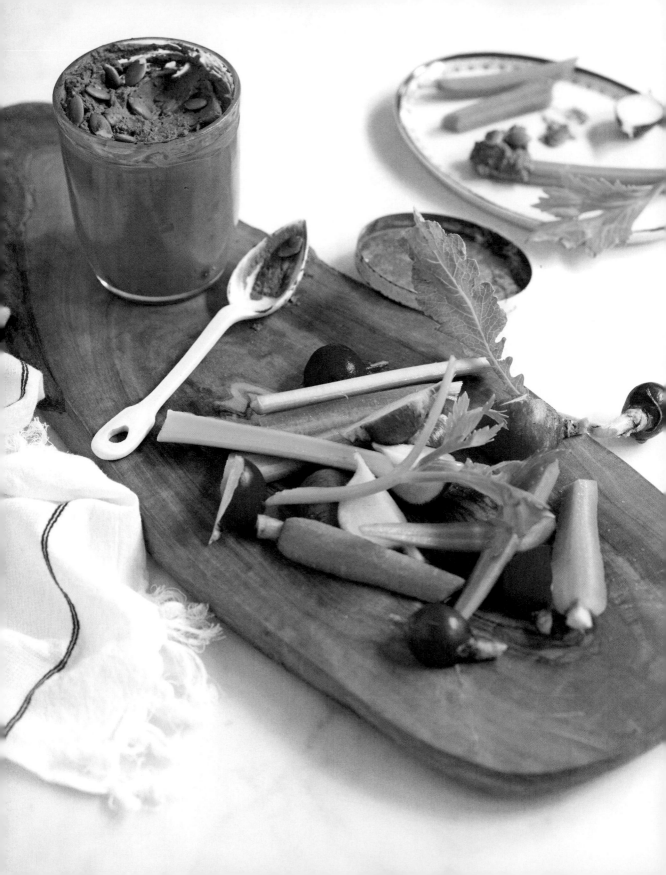

Creamy Marsala Wine Pâté Served with Crudités MAKES 2 JARS; 8 SERVINGS

Creamy pâté is the perfect party food, and also makes an ideal addition to an upscale picnic. It's a great showcase for organ meats, which are the most nutrient-dense cuts of the animal and are inexpensive. The liver is where B_{12} is stored, and it contains a staggering density of B vitamins. Try this recipe out on those who are new to eating liver, as the Marsala wine cuts the gamey taste liver can have.

- 1½ pounds chicken livers
- 1 teaspoon salt
- 4 tablespoons unsalted grass-fed butter, cubed
- 4 garlic cloves, minced
- ½ cup Marsala wine or bone broth (see page 200)
- ¼ cup pumpkin seeds
- 4 carrots, peeled and cut into matchsticks
- 4 celery stalks, cut into matchsticks
- ½ pound radishes, quartered

Line a plate with paper towels.

Trim the chicken livers of excess fat and sinew. Place in a colander and rinse under cold running water. Transfer to the paper towel–lined plate and dab excess moisture from the tops of the livers with another paper towel. Sprinkle with the salt.

Warm the butter in a large skillet over medium heat for about 30 seconds until it foams. Add the livers and garlic, and cook for 5 to 6 minutes until they start to brown and the garlic becomes fragrant. Carefully add the Marsala or broth and cook for 1 minute more, or until the livers are no longer bright red in the center but still pink. Remove from the heat and allow the livers to cool in the skillet for 5 minutes.

Transfer half the livers to a food processor and process until creamy and smooth,

about 30 seconds. Chop the remaining livers and stir in. Transfer the pâté to two glass airtight containers and sprinkle the pumpkin seeds on top, dividing them equally between the containers. Transfer to the fridge and chill the pâté for at least 1 hour before serving.

Serve with carrots, celery stalks, and radishes for dipping. Leftovers will keep for 5 days in the fridge.

NUTRITIONAL STATS PER SERVING (¼ POUND PÂTÉ WITH CRUDITÉS): 226 Calories ❖ 21g Protein ❖ 7g Carbohydrates ❖ 13g Fat (5g Saturated) ❖ 308mg Cholesterol ❖ 3g Sugars ❖ 3g Fiber ❖ 402mg Sodium

Vitamin B_{12} = 583% ❖ Vitamin A = 444% ❖ Folate = 136% ❖ Selenium = 87% ❖ Choline = 40%

Clove-Spiked Cocktail Nut Mix MAKES 3½ CUPS

Nuts are an ideal food: nutrient dense, easy to transport, and enjoyable to eat. Spices provide a free pass to flavor, since they are so low in calories—with only 3 to 4 calories per teaspoon, you can create sensational tastes. Zingy clove, the dried flower bud of an evergreen, is a warming spice used in traditional medicines and in cuisines around the world. Go easy on the Brazil nuts, though, as they are very high in selenium; you should not eat more than a few at a sitting to prevent selenium toxicity.

1 tablespoon olive oil
1 cup almonds
1 cup cashews
1 cup walnuts

½ cup Brazil nuts
1 teaspoon brown sugar
¾ teaspoon ground cloves

½ teaspoon freshly ground
   black pepper
½ teaspoon garlic salt
1 tablespoon water

Warm the olive oil in a medium skillet over medium heat. Add the almonds, cashews, walnuts, and Brazil nuts. Reduce the heat to low and cook for 2 to 3 minutes, stirring occasionally, until the nuts are fragrant. Sprinkle with the brown sugar, cloves, pepper, and garlic salt, and toss well. Drizzle with the water and stir well. Remove from the heat and allow to cool completely in the pan.

Store in an airtight container on the countertop up to 2 weeks.

NUTRITIONAL STATS PER SERVING (¼ CUP): 210
Calories ❖ 5g Protein ❖ 7g Carbohydrates ❖
19g Fat (2g Saturated) ❖ 0mg Cholesterol ❖
1g Sugars ❖ 2g Fiber ❖ 36mg Sodium

Selenium = 169% ❖ ALA = 71% ❖ Vitamin E = 40% ❖
Magnesium = 26% ❖ Zinc = 16%

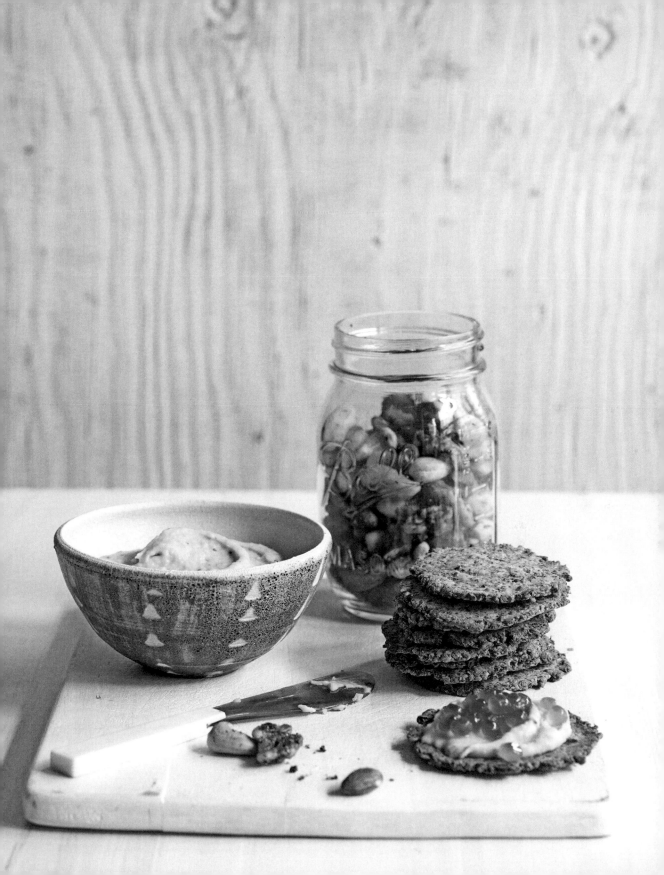

Sunflower-Parmesan Crisps with Navy Bean–Rosemary Hummus SERVES 8

Upgrade your cheese and crackers to a snack that's crunchy, delicious, and nutritious. These savory crisps are surprisingly simple to make, and fish roe is so nutrient dense that it needs a place in your food plan beyond the occasional appearance with sushi. Make an extra batch of the crackers to use as a snack, which you can dip in leftover red bell pepper coulis (page 124), or top with a thin slice of avocado or any of the pestos (pages 214 and 245) in this book.

½ cup olive oil, plus more for coating the baking sheet
½ cup sunflower seeds
½ cup ground flaxseeds
1 cup grated Parmesan cheese

2 egg whites, preferably from pasture-raised eggs
2 garlic cloves, halved
1 tablespoon fresh rosemary needles
1 teaspoon paprika

One 15.5-ounce can navy beans, rinsed well under cold running water and drained
1 cup fish eggs, such as salmon roe

Preheat the oven to 400°F. Coat a baking sheet with olive oil.

Put the sunflower seeds and flaxseeds in a food processor and pulse 8 to 10 times until the sunflower seeds are finely chopped. Add the Parmesan and egg whites and pulse 3 to 4 times until a thick batter forms. Drop the sunflower seed mixture onto the prepared baking sheet in scant tablespoon amounts, and press the tops down with a fork (you should have 24 crackers). Bake for 10 to 12 minutes until the crackers are lightly brown around the edges. Transfer to a plate to cool completely.

Place the garlic, rosemary, and paprika in the food processor and process until finely chopped. Add the beans and pulse 8 to 10 times until chunky. With the motor running, drizzle in the ½ cup olive oil and let the machine run until a thick creamy mixture forms.

For each serving, set out 3 crackers and top each with a heaping tablespoon of the hummus and a teaspoon of the fish eggs.

NUTRITIONAL STATS PER SERVING (3 CRACKERS TOPPED WITH HUMMUS AND FISH EGGS): 370 Calories ❖ 19g Protein ❖ 17g Carbohydrates ❖ 26g Fat (4g Saturated) ❖ 113mg Cholesterol ❖ 0g Sugars ❖ 6g Fiber ❖ 439mg Sodium

ALA = 137% ❖ Vitamin B$_{12}$ = 125% ❖ DHA+EPA = 120% ❖ Vitamin D = 67% ❖ Selenium = 42%

Sweet Potato Chips with Romesco Sauce SERVES 6

Upgrade the chip and the dip. Romesco is a tangy, creamy red pepper sauce, thickened with almonds and grilled bread, that hails from Spain. This gluten-free version uses oats in place of bread and is served with sweet potato in place of the traditional seafood pairing. If you have leftover sauce, serve it alongside cooked shrimp or your favorite flaky white fish.

2 red bell peppers

1 medium tomato, cored and quartered

¼ cup old-fashioned rolled oats

¼ cup whole almonds

2 tablespoons red wine vinegar

6 tablespoons olive oil

2 medium garlic cloves, peeled

½ teaspoon smoked paprika

¼ teaspoon salt

4 sweet potatoes (about 20 ounces), scrubbed

¼ teaspoon seasoning salt such as reduced-sodium Old Bay

Place the bell peppers on a baking sheet lined with aluminum foil. Place under the broiler and broil for 4 to 5 minutes, turning often, until the skins have blackened. Transfer the peppers to a bowl, cover with plastic wrap, and allow to steam for 5 minutes until the skins loosen. Remove and discard the skins, seeds, and stems.

Place the bell peppers, tomato, oats, almonds, vinegar, 4 tablespoons of the olive oil, the garlic, paprika, and salt in a food processor and process until a thick paste forms. Set aside.

Using a mandolin, thinly slice the sweet potatoes and transfer them to a large bowl. Toss the slices with the remaining 2 tablespoons of the olive oil and the seasoning salt. Spread the slices out in a single layer on a baking sheet and bake for 20 to 25 minutes, or until crisp. Serve immediately with the romesco sauce.

NUTRITIONAL STATS PER SERVING (30 CHIPS WITH ⅓ CUP ROMESCO): 259 Calories ❖ 4g Protein ❖ 25g Carbohydrates ❖ 17g Fat (2g Saturated) ❖ 0mg Cholesterol ❖ 6g Sugars ❖ 5g Fiber ❖ 180mg Sodium

Vitamin A = 98% ❖ Vitamin C = 75% ❖ Fiber = 20% ❖ Magnesium = 17% ❖ Vitamin K = 14%

Citrus Scallops with Spinach, Asparagus, and Marinated Kirby Cucumber SERVES 4

Citrus and spice combine to make this a great dish for seafood lovers and newbies alike. Scallops are very accessible, as they are mild and simple to prepare—whether cooked or raw as in a ceviche (page 250). Turmeric, a rhizome related to ginger, has anti-inflammatory properties and is one of the few compounds known to increase BDNF, a regulator of brain connections.

4 Kirby cucumbers, thinly sliced

2 tablespoons raw apple cider vinegar

¼ teaspoon salt

2 pounds baby spinach

2 large oranges

1 pound dry (untreated) sea scallops

½ teaspoon paprika

¼ teaspoon ground turmeric

¼ teaspoon freshly ground black pepper

2 tablespoons coconut oil

1 pound asparagus, trimmed and chopped

3 tablespoons balsamic vinegar

Combine the cucumbers, vinegar, and salt in a large bowl and toss well. Divide the spinach among four large dinner plates and top with the cucumbers.

Using a microplane, finely grate the zest of the oranges onto a plate. Working over a medium bowl to catch the juices, cut the oranges into segments and set aside.

Sprinkle the scallops with the orange zest, paprika, turmeric, and pepper. Warm 1 tablespoon of the coconut oil in a large skillet over medium-high heat. Add the scallops and sear for 3 to 4 minutes, turning once, until the scallops start to brown and are no longer translucent in the center. Transfer the scallops to the salad plates, distributing them equally.

Add the remaining 1 tablespoon coconut oil and the asparagus to the skillet in which you cooked the scallops. Cook the asparagus pieces over medium heat for 1 to 2 minutes until they start to turn a darker shade of green but are still crisp. Turn off the heat, add the balsamic vinegar, and stir well. Divide the asparagus equally among the dinner plates and top with the orange segments. Serve immediately.

NUTRITIONAL STATS PER SERVING: 334 Calories ❖ 24g Protein ❖ 37g Carbohydrates ❖ 11g Fat (9g Saturated) ❖ 27mg Cholesterol ❖ 16g Sugars ❖ 11g Fiber ❖ 774mg Sodium

Vitamin K = 1,317% ❖ Vitamin A = 163% ❖ Vitamin C = 152% ❖ Folate = 136% ❖ Iodine = 90%

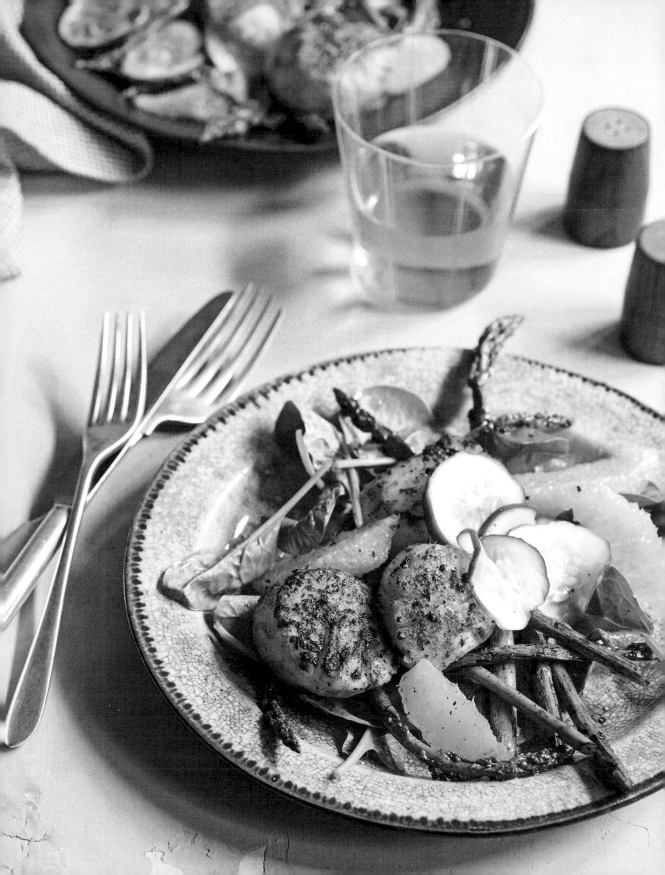

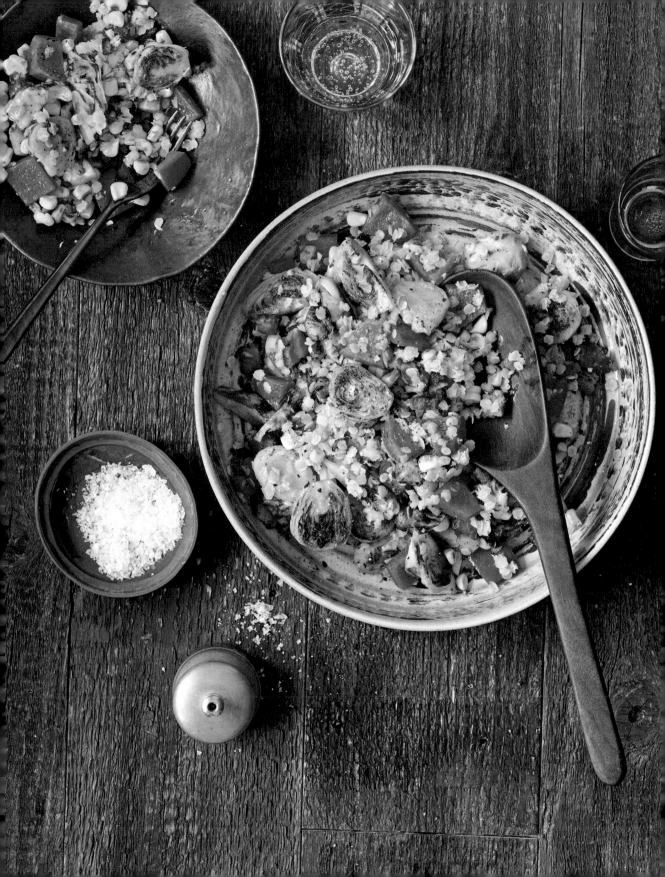

Pancetta Brussels Sprouts with Red Lentil Succotash SERVES 4

Long abused, boiled, and received with frowns, the Brussels sprout is finally having its moment. Still, eating more plants and plant proteins can be a challenge for many meat lovers. Enter pancetta, which can add to the appeal of any vegetable. Lentils are a top source of folate and should be a diet staple, as they are simple, inexpensive, and nutritious. This colorful dish makes great use of the late summer and early fall harvest at your local farmers' market, so stock up on fresh corn and bell peppers. For spice lovers, sprinkle ½ teaspoon of ground cayenne to add a bit of heat, or add a small seeded and chopped jalapeño.

1 cup uncooked red lentils
1 tablespoon olive oil
4 ounces chopped pancetta

1 pound Brussels sprouts, trimmed and quartered
1 red bell pepper, seeded and chopped
2 garlic cloves, minced

1 cup fresh corn kernels, or defrosted frozen corn kernels
Garlic salt
Freshly ground black pepper

Cook the lentils according to the package instructions, drain, and set aside.

Coat a large skillet with olive oil and place it over medium-high heat. Add the pancetta and cook for 1 to 2 minutes, stirring often, until it starts to brown. Reduce the heat to medium-low, and continue to cook the pancetta until crispy. Using a slotted spoon, transfer the pancetta to a bowl. Do not discard the fat in the pan; you will use it to cook the vegetables.

Place the skillet containing the fat over medium heat. Add the Brussels sprouts and cook for 3 to 4 minutes, turning often, until they begin to brown. Reduce the heat to low and add the bell pepper and garlic.

Cook for 3 to 4 minutes more, stirring occasionally, until the sprouts are tender and the bell pepper is cooked through. Add the corn and reserved lentils, sprinkle with the garlic salt and black pepper, and cook for 1 minute more. Serve immediately.

NUTRITIONAL STATS PER SERVING (2 CUPS): 359 Calories ❖ 22g Protein ❖ 49g Carbohydrates ❖ 9g Fat (3g Saturated) ❖ 10mg Cholesterol ❖ 7g Sugars ❖ 20g Fiber ❖ 315mg Sodium

Vitamin K = 228% ❖ Vitamin C = 187% ❖ Folate = 82% ❖ Fiber = 81% ❖ Protein = 50%

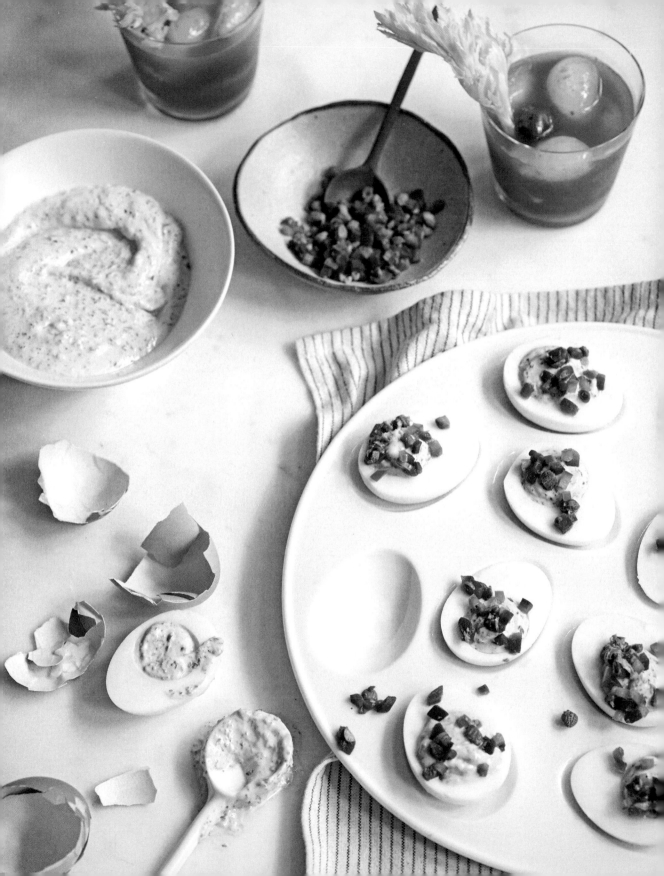

Deviled Green Eggs with Roasted Red Pepper and Capers SERVES 4

Deviled eggs are always a crowd-pleaser and are a great way to extend your relationship with eggs beyond breakfast. Here's a twist on the classic that packs more flavor and far more nutrition with the powers of mustard greens and roasted red pepper. These are great for a snack or for lunch at work. If you prefer to roast the peppers yourself, place them on a baking sheet under the broiler for 3 to 4 minutes, turning often, until the skins are blackened. Transfer to a bowl and let them steam for 5 minutes. Then peel and seed the peppers before completing the recipe.

8 pasture-raised eggs

1 teaspoon white vinegar

1 cup trimmed mustard greens

½ cup olive oil–based mayonnaise

¼ teaspoon freshly ground black pepper

¼ cup diced roasted red peppers

2 tablespoons capers, rinsed and chopped

1 jalapeño, seeded and minced (optional)

Put the eggs and vinegar in a small saucepan and cover with cold water. Bring to a full boil over high heat, cover, and turn off the heat. Set aside for 15 minutes to allow the eggs to cook through. Place under cold running water to cool. Drain and peel. Cut the eggs in half lengthwise, scoop out the yolks, and transfer them to a small bowl. Set aside.

Put the mustard greens in a food processor and chop finely. Add the reserved egg yolks, mayonnaise, and black pepper and process until smooth. Transfer the egg whites to a plate and fill them with the yolk mixture. Top with the roasted red peppers,

capers, and jalapeño, if using. Serve immediately, or cover and chill until ready to serve or for up to 4 hours.

NUTRITIONAL STATS PER SERVING (4 PIECES):
255 Calories ❖ 13g Protein ❖ 4g Carbohydrates ❖ 19g Fat (4g Saturated) ❖ 382mg Cholesterol ❖ 1g Sugars ❖ 1g Fiber ❖ 555mg Sodium

Vitamin K = 157% ❖ Choline = 69% ❖ Selenium = 56% ❖ Vitamin A = 46% ❖ Vitamin D = 40%

Chicken Satay with Peanut–Pumpkin Seed Dipping Sauce SERVES 4

This small plate has serious appeal to kids, with a creamy dipping sauce that will have them cheering. Parents will be cheering, too, for the zinc and magnesium found in the pumpkin seeds that help build smarter, happier brains. If your youngsters can't do peanuts, use almonds or pecans instead. For an extra brain boost, sprinkle the chicken with ¼ teaspoon ground turmeric.

½ cup peanuts

¼ cup pumpkin seeds

¼ cup canned coconut milk

2 tablespoons reduced-sodium soy sauce

2 garlic cloves

2 teaspoons hot sauce (optional)

¼ cup fresh Thai basil, chopped (optional)

2 large boneless, skinless chicken breasts (about ¾ pound)

Twelve 6-inch skewers, soaked for 30 minutes in cold water

1 tablespoon coconut oil

½ teaspoon chili powder, mild or hot

¼ teaspoon freshly ground black pepper

½ pound raw green beans, stems removed

Place the peanuts, pumpkin seeds, coconut milk, soy sauce, garlic, and hot sauce, if using, in a food processor or mini chopper. Blend until smooth, adding a few tablespoons of water to adjust consistency until creamy if needed. Sprinkle with the chopped basil, if using, and set the satay sauce aside.

Cut each chicken breast into eight 4-inch-long strips (for a total of 16 strips). Thread the chicken onto the soaked bamboo skewers and rub with the coconut oil. Season the skewered chicken on both sides with the chili powder and black pepper.

Preheat a grill to medium-high heat. Grill the skewered chicken for 3 to 4 minutes per side, for a total of 6 to 8 minutes, until it is cooked through. Serve immediately with the satay sauce and green beans.

NUTRITIONAL STATS PER SERVING (4 SKEWERS AND ¼ CUP SAUCE): 360 Calories ❖ 29g Protein ❖ 11g Carbohydrates ❖ 24g Fat (6g Saturated) ❖ 54mg Cholesterol ❖ 1g Sugars ❖ 3g Fiber ❖ 433mg Sodium

Protein = 62% ❖ Selenium = 53% ❖ Magnesium = 37% ❖ Zinc = 23% ❖ Vitamin C = 19%

Grains

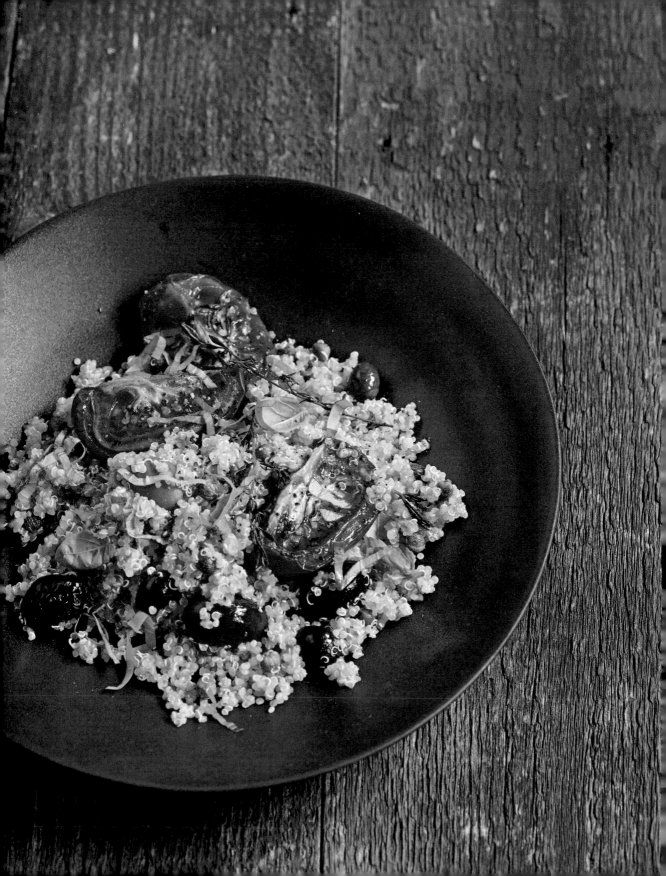

Warm Herby Quinoa with Tomato Confit, Olives, and Capers SERVES 4

This savory Mediterranean-inspired dish can make for a luscious summer meal served alongside a simple green salad or grilled zucchini and eggplant (page 178). For wine pairings, search out lemony sauvignon blancs or fruitier New World pinot noirs. To make this salad "finger friendly," hollow out cucumber halves and fill with the salad.

1 pound tomatoes, quartered

1 tablespoon olive oil

1 teaspoon fresh thyme leaves

½ teaspoon salt

¼ teaspoon freshly ground black pepper

1 cup red or white quinoa

½ cup assorted olives, packed in oil

¼ cup capers, rinsed well and drained

2 tablespoons tomato paste

½ cup torn fresh basil leaves

Preheat the oven to 250°F.

Arrange the tomatoes, cut side up, on a large baking sheet. Drizzle with the olive oil and sprinkle with the thyme leaves, salt, and pepper. Transfer to the oven and bake for about 1 hour, turning once or twice, until the tomatoes have shrunk and are lightly browned.

Cook the quinoa according to the package instructions, then toss with the olives, capers, and tomato paste. Transfer the quinoa to a platter and spoon the tomatoes over it. Sprinkle with the basil and serve immediately.

NUTRITIONAL STATS PER SERVING (2 CUPS): 236 Calories ❖ 8g Protein ❖ 35g Carbohydrates ❖ 8g Fat (1g Saturated) ❖ 0mg Cholesterol ❖ 4g Sugars ❖ 6g Fiber ❖ 682mg Sodium

Vitamin C = 41% ❖ Selenium = 33% ❖ Calcium = 28% ❖ Fiber = 24% ❖ Vitamin D = 21%

Quinoa can be cooked ahead of time, so make a double batch to use for several of the recipes in the book. Cool it completely before storing in an airtight container, refrigerated, for up to 5 days, or in the freezer for up to 6 weeks.

Black Rice with Grilled Radicchio, Beets, and Goat Cheese SERVES 4

This vegetarian feast from the grill will add health to any cookout. You may be surprised by the idea of beets on the grill, but grilling is easier than boiling them, and placing them in aluminum foil speeds the process. To add grill marks to the beets, remove them from the foil during the last 5 minutes of grilling and put them in a grilling basket or grill them directly on grates.

1 cup black rice
1 pound beets with tops: beets peeled and quartered, tops (½ pound) reserved
3 tablespoons olive oil

¼ cup chopped fresh herbs such as chives, basil, or parsley
2 tablespoons raw apple cider vinegar
1 tablespoon tomato paste

1 tablespoon water
½ pound radicchio, quartered
8 ounces soft goat cheese or Brie

Cook the black rice according to the package instructions. Preheat a grill over high heat.

Cut the tops off the beets. Wash and dry the beet greens, place them in a bowl, and reserve. Mix the quartered beets with 1 tablespoon olive oil and wrap them in aluminum foil. Place them on the preheated grill and cook for 40 to 45 minutes until tender.

While the beets are cooking, prepare the dressing. Place the herbs, the remaining 2 tablespoons olive oil, the vinegar, and the tomato paste in a bowl along with the water. Stir well to combine and set aside.

When the beets are cooked, place the radicchio on the grill for 2 to 3 minutes until charred and tender. Wilt the reserved beet greens by placing them on the grill for 1 minute. Arrange the beet greens on a platter. Slice the radicchio and arrange it over the greens. Scatter the beets on top of the greens and spoon the rice over them. Dot with the goat cheese or Brie. Drizzle with the dressing and serve immediately.

NUTRITIONAL STATS PER SERVING (2½ CUPS SALAD): 454 Calories ❖ 19g Protein ❖ 51g Carbohydrates ❖ 20g Fat (9g Saturated) ❖ 26mg Cholesterol ❖ 9g Sugars ❖ 6g Fiber ❖ 471mg Sodium

Vitamin K = 427% ❖ ALA = 120% ❖ Vitamin A = 51% ❖ Folate = 44% ❖ Protein = 41%

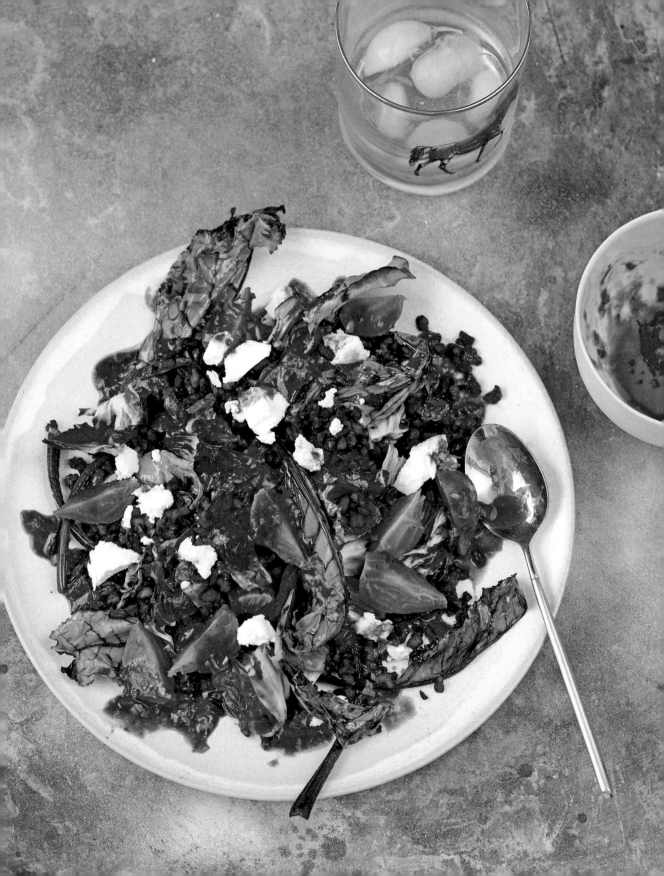

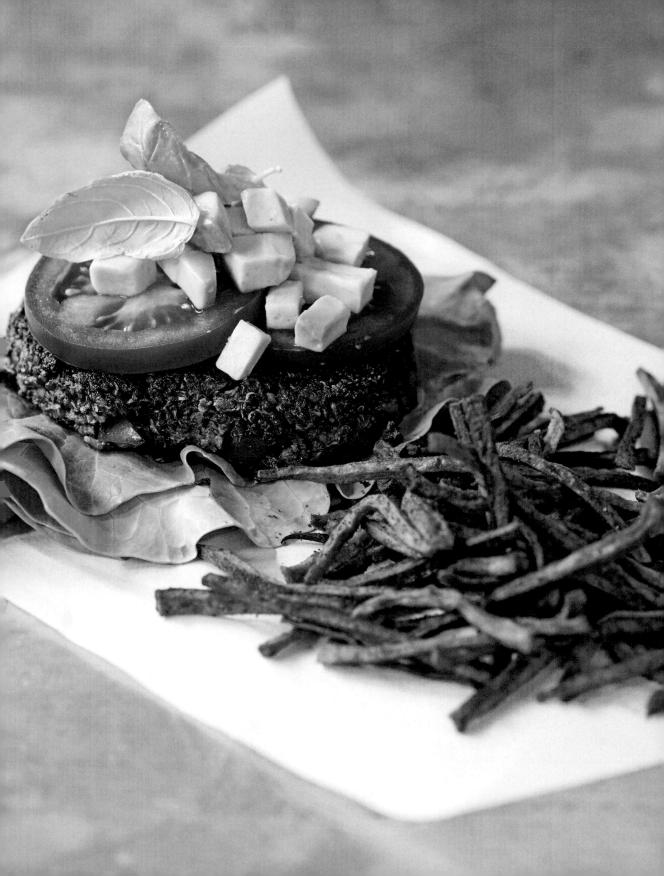

Rainbow Burgers with Golden Turmeric Sweet Potato Fries SERVES 4

This plant-based burger contains twelve different nutrient-dense plants. Eat the rainbow with one serving of this dish, which provides a wide array of nutrients and phytonutrients all on one plate. As a shortcut, you can substitute good-quality frozen sweet potato fries instead of the fresh version—just be sure they are made with a preferred fat such as olive oil.

½ cup uncooked white or red quinoa

2 cups kale or watercress

¼ red onion, quartered

½ cup fresh cilantro or dill

One 15-ounce can low-sodium black beans, rinsed well under cold running water and drained

1 pasture-raised egg

1 red bell pepper, seeded and diced

4 sweet potatoes, peeled and cut into matchsticks

4 tablespoons safflower or coconut oil

½ teaspoon paprika

½ teaspoon chipotle chile powder or mild chili powder

¼ teaspoon ground turmeric

¼ teaspoon salt

4 large collard leaves, well washed and trimmed

1 avocado, pitted, peeled, and sliced

Cook the quinoa according to the package instructions and set aside.

Place the kale or watercress, onion, and cilantro or dill in a food processor and pulse 8 to 10 times to roughly chop. Add the quinoa and the beans, and pulse until a chunky mixture forms. Stir in the egg and diced bell pepper. Form the mixture into four 4-inch-diameter burgers and place on a plate. Chill the burgers for 30 minutes.

Preheat oven to 400°F. Prepare the fries. Toss the potatoes in a large bowl along with half the oil, the paprika, chipotle or chili powder, turmeric, and salt. Spread out the fries on two ungreased baking sheets. Bake for 25 to 30 minutes, turning occasionally, until browned and fork-tender.

While the fries are baking, cook the burgers. Warm the remaining oil in a large skillet over medium-high heat. Add the burgers and cook for 4 to 5 minutes, turning once or twice, until they are well browned. Transfer the burgers to the collard leaves, top with the avocado slices, and serve immediately with the fries.

NUTRITIONAL STATS PER SERVING (1 BURGER WITH FRIES): 458 Calories ❖ 14g Protein ❖ 68g Carbohydrates ❖ 17g Fat (2g Saturated) ❖ 46mg Cholesterol ❖ 8g Sugars ❖ 17g Fiber ❖ 472mg Sodium

Vitamin K = 250% ❖ Vitamin A = 168% ❖ Vitamin C = 152% ❖ Fiber = 68% ❖ Folate = 43%

Lazy Green Mac and Cheese SERVES 4

Simple and nutritious, this dish is a great way to get more greens on the table, and is an antidote to carbohydrate cravings. Whole grain quinoa pasta is a good start, but the nutrient density of this dish soars thanks to the addition of the greens, which bring significant amounts of vitamin K, vitamin A, and vitamin C. It takes under 20 minutes to make, and kids devour it. It's best eaten right out of the oven when the cheese is bubbling and hot.

Olive oil

8 ounces quinoa pasta, such as elbows, penne, or shells

½ pound mustard greens or kale, trimmed and chopped (3 to 4 cups)

1½ cups grated cheddar cheese

Preheat the oven to 400°F. Coat a 7 × 11-inch dish with olive oil.

Cook the quinoa pasta according to the package instructions. Drain the pasta and spread it out in the prepared dish. Sprinkle with the chopped greens and cheese, and transfer to the oven. Bake for 15 to 20 minutes until the cheese has melted and is bubbling hot.

NUTRITIONAL STATS PER SERVING (2 CUPS): 443
Calories ❖ 19g Protein ❖ 52g Carbohydrates ❖
18g Fat (11g Saturated) ❖ 51mg Cholesterol ❖
2g Sugars ❖ 5g Fiber ❖ 343mg Sodium

Vitamin K = 516% ❖ Vitamin C = 91% ❖
Vitamin A = 84% ❖ Protein = 41% ❖ Calcium = 40%

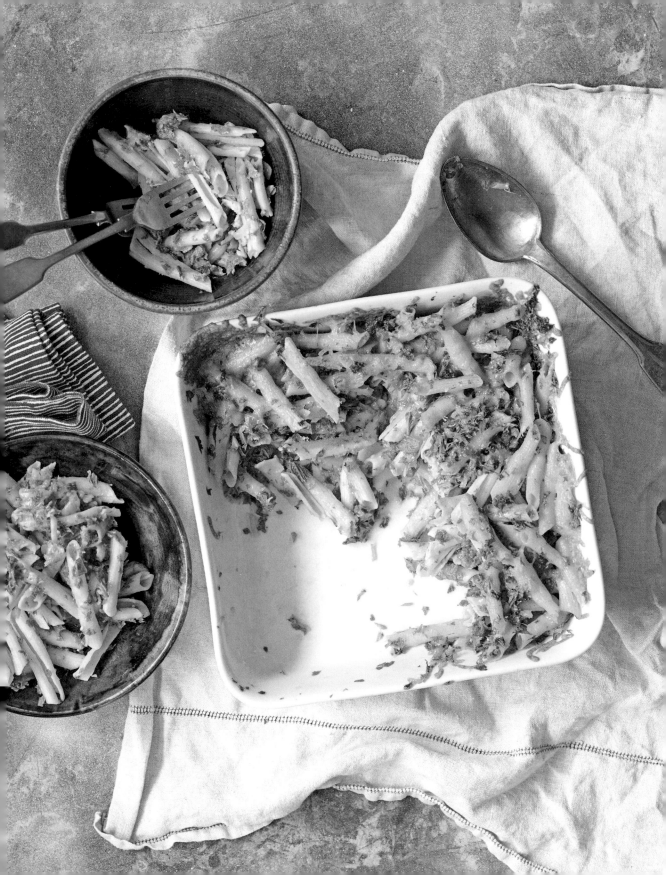

Sweet and Sour Brussels Sprouts SERVES 4

Tomato and grapefruit make up the sweet and sour sauce of this eye-catching dish that is ideal for brunch or as part of a tapas menu. Cruciferous Brussels sprouts promote health with phyonutrients, vitamin K, and vitamin C, and they help boost your mood with folate. Serve as a side with roasted chicken or baked fresh fish, or toss it with sautéed shrimp or strips of beef to turn it into a main meal.

½ cup uncooked millet or quinoa

1 pink or ruby grapefruit

2 tablespoons coconut oil

2 pints Brussels sprouts, trimmed and halved

½ teaspoon salt

2 tablespoons tomato paste

½ teaspoon Dijon mustard

Cook the millet or quinoa according to the package instructions and set aside.

Using a sharp knife, cut away the grapefruit peel and white pith. Working over a bowl, cut the grapefruit into segments, allowing any juice to fall into the bowl.

Heat a large, oven-safe skillet over medium-high heat. Add the coconut oil and the Brussels sprouts and cook for 2 to 3 minutes without moving them, or until the Brussels sprouts start to brown. Turn the sprouts over and transfer the skillet to the middle rack of the oven. Turn on the broiler and broil for 20 minutes until the tops are brown.

Transfer the millet to a platter and top with the Brussels sprouts.

In the skillet in which you cooked the Brussels sprouts, whisk together the reserved grapefruit juice, salt, tomato

paste, and mustard. Toss in the grapefruit segments. Spoon the mixture over the Brussels sprouts and grains and serve immediately.

NUTRITIONAL STATS PER SERVING (2 CUPS): 231 Calories ❖ 7g Protein ❖ 33g Carbohydrates ❖ 8g Fat (6g Saturated) ❖ 0mg Cholesterol ❖ 8g Sugars ❖ 6g Fiber ❖ 640mg Sodium

Vitamin K = 174% ❖ Vitamin C = 128% ❖ Fiber, Thiamine = 24% ❖ Folate = 21% ❖ Magnesium = 18%

Amaranth Griddle Cakes with Tomato-Ginger Chutney SERVES 4

Tomato, lemon, and ginger are a delectable trio that you'll find in sauces and chutneys of traditional Indian cuisine. All three offer the benefits of phytonutrients: the fat-protecting lycopene in tomatoes, the pleasure-inducing and inflammation-fighting liminoids in lemon, and the anticancer gingerols in ginger. Frankly, your daily medicine never tasted better.

½ cup uncooked amaranth
1¼ cups water
3 tablespoons coconut oil
One 2-inch piece fresh ginger, peeled and minced
½ lemon, diced (including the rind), seeds removed
1 pound tomatoes, chopped
1 red bell pepper, seeded and minced
¾ cup unsweetened shredded coconut
4 thinly sliced scallions
2 large pasture-raised eggs
¼ cup pumpkin seeds, roughly chopped
1 teaspoon baking powder
¼ teaspoon salt

Put the amaranth and water in a saucepan and cook for 15 to 20 minutes until the amaranth is tender and a thick porridge forms. Transfer the amaranth to a large bowl and let cool for 5 minutes.

Prepare the chutney. Warm 1 tablespoon of the coconut oil in a small saucepan over medium heat. Add the ginger and lemon and cook for 3 to 4 minutes until the lemon starts to brown. Add the tomatoes and reduce the heat to low and simmer for 10 to 15 minutes.

Add the coconut, scallions, eggs, pumpkin seeds, baking powder, and salt to the cooled amaranth and stir well.

Warm a large cast-iron skillet or griddle over medium heat. Add 1 tablespoon of oil. Working in two batches, drop 6 mounds

of the batter (about ¼ cup each) into the hot skillet and cook for 3 to 4 minutes until the edges are firm and the cakes are well browned. Flip and cook for 3 minutes more until the cakes are firm. Transfer the cakes to a plate. Add the remaining 1 tablespoon oil to the skillet before cooking the second batch.

Set out four plates and top each with 3 cakes. Spoon the chutney over the cakes and serve immediately.

NUTRITIONAL STATS PER SERVING (3 CAKES WITH 2 TABLESPOONS SAUCE): 292 Calories ❖ 10g Protein ❖ 27g Carbohydrates ❖ 17g Fat (9g Saturated) ❖ 93mg Cholesterol ❖ 6g Sugars ❖ 5g Fiber ❖ 286mg Sodium

Vitamin C = 77% ❖ Vitamin K = 47% ❖ Magnesium = 42% ❖ Zinc, Selenium = 25% ❖ Protein = 22%

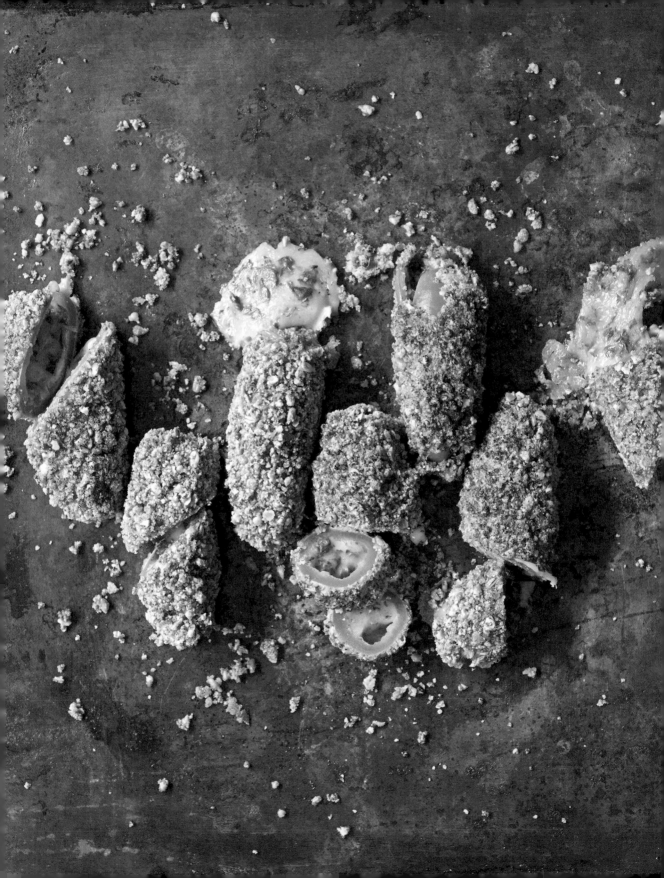

Millet-Jalapeño Poppers SERVES 4

Jalapeño poppers from a bar menu or in the freezer aisle don't have much in the way of nutrition. But making them yourself is quite easy, and using fresh jalapeños means more flavor and improved texture. Thanks to the spinach, millet, and sunflower seeds, these poppers provide a bevy of nutrients like vitamin C, zinc, and folate.

8 large jalapeños

4 cups fresh spinach leaves, chopped

2 pasture-raised eggs

½ cup cooked millet

⅓ cup sunflower seeds

2 tablespoons ground flaxseeds

1 cup grated cheddar cheese

Olive oil cooking spray or mister

½ teaspoon seasoning salt such as reduced-sodium Old Bay

Preheat the oven to 400°F.

Cut the stem ends off the jalapeños. Using a melon baller, scoop out the seeds.

Warm a large skillet over high heat. Put in the spinach and cook for 1 minute until wilted. Set aside.

Crack the eggs into a shallow dish and whisk gently with a fork.

Place the millet, sunflower seeds, and ground flaxseeds in a food processor and pulse until a fine meal forms. Transfer the mixture to a plate.

Stuff each jalapeño with 2 tablespoons of the cheese and the spinach. Roll the jalapeños in the egg, then press firmly into the millet mixture.

Transfer the jalapeños to a baking sheet. Coat the tops with olive oil (spray or mist) and bake for 8 to 10 minutes until the cheese starts to ooze out. Sprinkle with the seasoning salt, cool 5 minutes, and serve.

NUTRITIONAL STATS PER SERVING (2 PIECES):
280 Calories ❖ 14g Protein ❖ 14g Carbohydrates ❖ 18g Fat (7g Saturated) ❖ 122mg Cholesterol ❖ 1g Sugars ❖ 3g Fiber ❖ 358mg Sodium

Vitamin K = 159% ❖ Vitamin C = 55% ❖ Vitamin A and Selenium = 38% ❖ Protein = 30% ❖ Folate, Zinc = 28%

Baked Creamy Quinoa Casserole with Asparagus and Artichokes SERVES 6

Creamy and satisfying, this dish channels the ubiquitous green bean casserole and has the same comfort food appeal while packing a nutritious punch. If you're preparing this for the holidays or a special occasion, you can prep it ahead of time. Mix the cooked quinoa with the vegetables and the remaining ingredients, then store in the fridge until you're ready to bake.

1 cup uncooked red or white quinoa

1 pound asparagus, trimmed and chopped

1 cup artichoke hearts, chopped

1 cup olive oil–based mayonnaise

½ cup fresh basil leaves, measured, then chopped

½ cup grated pecorino Romano cheese

¼ cup cold water

1 teaspoon Dijon mustard

½ teaspoon paprika

1 teaspoon baking powder

Preheat the oven to 400°F.

Cook the quinoa according to the package instructions and cool 5 minutes. Transfer to a large bowl along with the asparagus, artichokes, mayonnaise, basil, cheese, and cold water. Stir well to combine, then mix in the mustard, paprika, and baking powder. Transfer to an 8 × 8-inch baking dish.

Bake for 20 to 25 minutes until hot and puffed, then cool 5 minutes before serving.

NUTRITIONAL STATS PER SERVING (1 CUP): 295
Calories ❖ 8g Protein ❖ 26g Carbohydrates ❖ 17g Fat (2g Saturated) ❖ 20mg Cholesterol ❖ 1g Sugars ❖ 6g Fiber ❖ 500mg Sodium

Vitamin K = 48% ❖ Choline = 37% ❖ Folate = 30% ❖ Fiber = 24% ❖ Thiamine = 21%

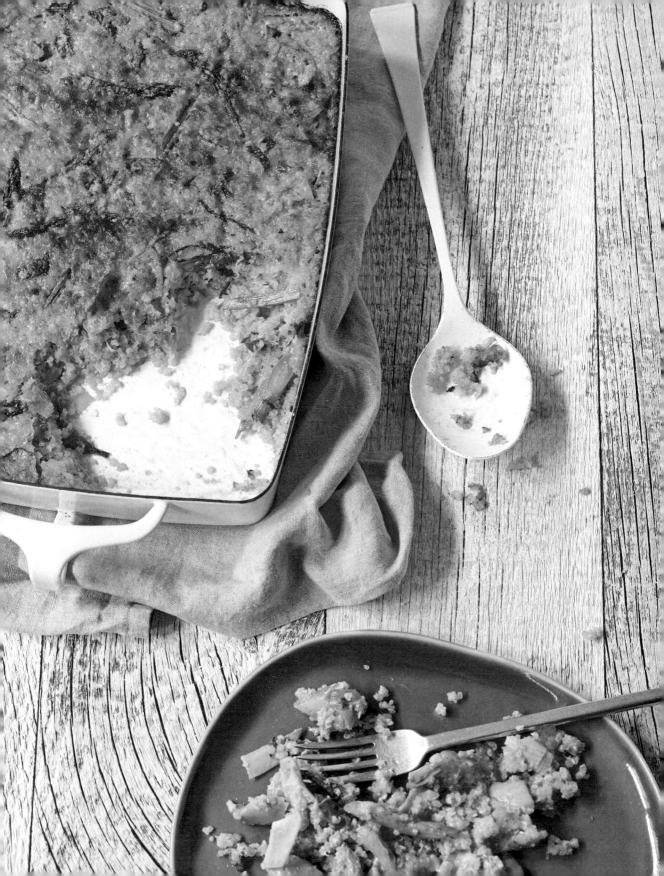

Love Grass with Radishes and Ramps SERVES 4

Teff—a tiny, nutty, quick-cooking grain that is also known as love grass—was one of the first domesticated grains. The small seeds of teff boast protein, calcium, and B vitamins. Melted havarti cheese mixed with cool radishes gives flavor and texture contrast to make this dish extra-special. If you can't find ramps, or want to substitute something for them, use baby leeks instead, and trim the tough greens, or opt for ½ pound of asparagus spears.

½ cup uncooked teff

1 cup low-sodium chicken stock or vegetable stock

½ cup cold water, plus 2 tablespoons

¼ teaspoon salt

2 tablespoons sour cream

2 tablespoons olive oil–based mayonnaise

¼ cup chopped fresh chives

4 radishes, trimmed and thinly sliced

8 ramps, thinly sliced

¼ cup chopped fresh tarragon or basil

1 cup grated havarti cheese

Place the teff in a medium stockpot along with the chicken or vegetable stock and the ½ cup cold water and bring to a boil over medium heat. Reduce the heat to low and simmer for 15 to 20 minutes until a thick porridge forms and the grains of teff are tender. Turn off the heat and set the teff aside.

Combine the salt, sour cream, and mayonnaise in a large bowl, along with the chives and the 2 tablespoons cold water and stir well. Add the radishes and ramps and toss to coat. Mix in the tarragon or basil. Transfer the mixture to an oven-safe platter or casserole dish, and spoon the teff over the top. Sprinkle with the havarti and place under the broiler for 30 seconds, or until the cheese has melted. Serve immediately.

NUTRITIONAL STATS PER SERVING (1½ CUPS):
248 Calories ❖ 11g Protein ❖ 23g Carbohydrates ❖ 13g Fat (7g Saturated) ❖ 30mg Cholesterol ❖ 2g Sugars ❖ 2g Fiber ❖ 489mg Sodium

Vitamin K = 36% ❖ Protein = 24% ❖ Magnesium = 17% ❖ Vitamin A = 14% ❖ Zinc = 13%

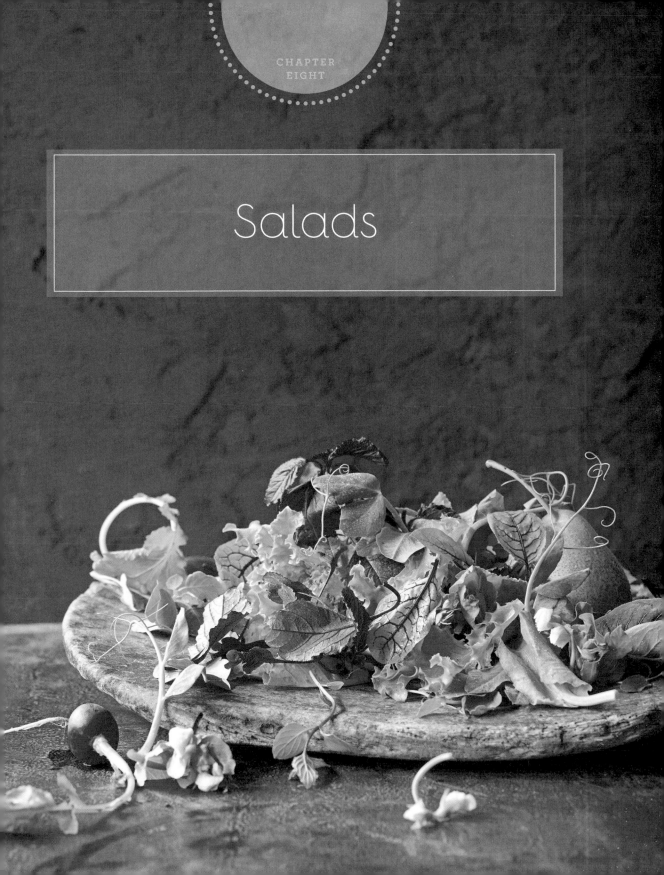

Salads

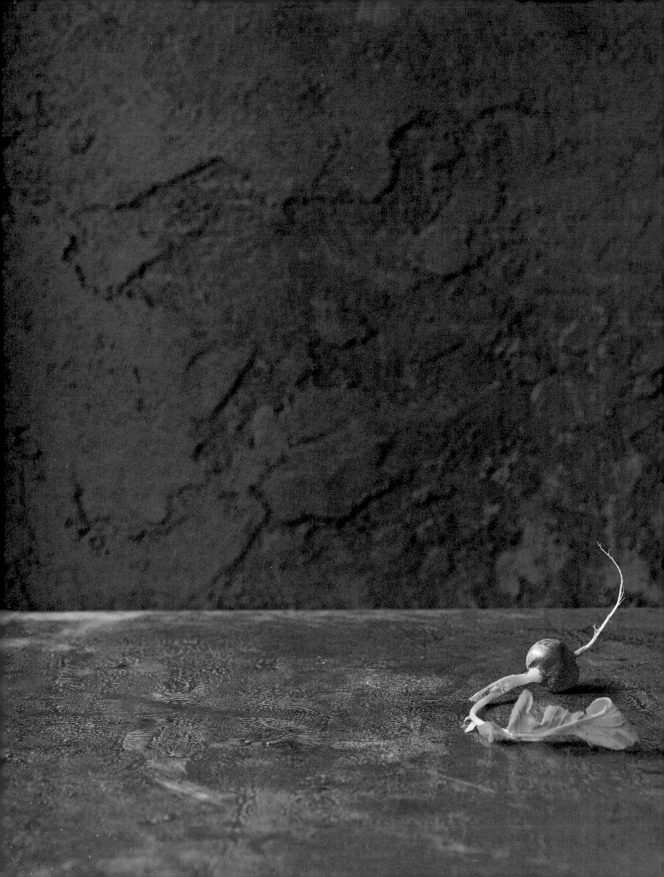

Hearty Winter Kale Salad with Roasted Purple Potatoes and Hemp Seeds SERVES 4

Revive your appreciation for potatoes and anchovies with this dish. Kale thrives in the fall and early winter, and has a sweeter taste as the temperature starts to drop. Potatoes are a good source of potassium and iodine. Purple potatoes are a healthy starch option and make this salad hearty and filling. If you can't find purple potatoes, you can use small Red Bliss or creamer potatoes in their place.

1 garlic clove

½ cup freshly grated Parmesan cheese

1 egg yolk, preferably from a pasture-raised egg

2 anchovies, minced

Juice of 1 lemon

2 tablespoons olive oil

¼ teaspoon freshly ground black pepper

One 10-ounce bunch kale, preferably lacinato, stems trimmed

2 tablespoons grass-fed butter or reserved bacon fat

½ pound purple potatoes, quartered

¼ teaspoon salt

¼ teaspoon freshly ground black pepper

2 tablespoons hemp seeds

Rub a mixing bowl with the garlic clove. Then combine the Parmesan, egg yolk, anchovies, lemon juice, olive oil, and black pepper in the bowl and whisk well. Tear the kale leaves and place them in the bowl along with the dressing. Squeeze the leaves with your fingers, crushing the kale to tenderize it while mixing with the dressing for about 1 minute. Cover the salad and set aside.

Warm the grass-fed butter or bacon fat in a cast-iron skillet over medium heat. Add the potatoes and season with the salt and pepper, stirring well. Cover and cook for 8 to 10 minutes, stirring occasionally, until the potatoes soften. Remove the lid and cook for 1 to 2 minutes more until the potatoes are crisp.

Divide the kale among four plates and top with the hot potatoes. Sprinkle with the hemp seeds and serve immediately.

NUTRITIONAL STATS PER SERVING (3 CUPS): 322 Calories ❖ 11g Protein ❖ 18g Carbohydrates ❖ 24g Fat (4g Saturated) ❖ 57mg Cholesterol ❖ 3g Sugars ❖ 3g Fiber ❖ 430mg Sodium

Vitamin K = 649% ❖ Vitamin C = 127% ❖ Vitamin A = 84% ❖ Protein = 24% ❖ Thiamine = 18%

Grilled Grass-Fed Beef and Watercress Salad with Avocado and Golden Beets SERVES 4

This dish is another doorway to plants for meat lovers, since it combines iron-rich flank steak with watercress, a heavy hitter when it comes to nutrients such as vitamins A, C, and K. Watercress is at its peak in the spring, but most grocery stores carry it throughout the summer months as well. If you can't find it, baby spinach will work as a substitute.

½ pound golden beets, peeled and quartered
1 tablespoon olive oil
1 pound grass-fed flank steak
¼ teaspoon salt
8 ounces watercress

1 ripe Hass avocado, pitted, peeled, and cubed
Dressing
3 tablespoons olive oil
3 tablespoons balsamic vinegar

1 tablespoon chopped fresh rosemary
2 teaspoons honey
1 teaspoon Dijon mustard
¼ teaspoon salt

Preheat a grill over high heat.

Mix the beets with the olive oil and place in a grill basket, or wrap in aluminum foil and place on the grill. Grill for 25 to 30 minutes until the beets are tender. During the last 5 minutes of cooking, transfer them directly to the grill for grill marks.

While the beets are cooking, prepare the steak. Place the flank steak on a plate and sprinkle with the salt. Grill the beef for 15 to 20 minutes, turning occasionally, until medium rare. Let the steak rest for 5 minutes to allow the juices to redistribute before slicing.

While the steak is resting, prepare the dressing. Put the olive oil, vinegar,

rosemary, honey, mustard, and salt in a small bowl and whisk well to combine.

Arrange the watercress on four plates and top with the beets and avocado, dividing them equally. Slice the steak into thin, ⅛-inch slices, and divide the slices among the four plates. Drizzle with the dressing and serve immediately.

NUTRITIONAL STATS PER SERVING: 412 Calories ❖ 28g Protein ❖ 21g Carbohydrate ❖ 24g Fat (6g Saturated) ❖ 21mg Cholesterol ❖ 14g Sugars ❖ 5g Fiber ❖ 470mg Sodium

Vitamin K = 184% ❖ Vitamin B$_{12}$ = 117% ❖ Zinc = 96% ❖ Selenium = 64% ❖ Protein, Vitamin C = 63%

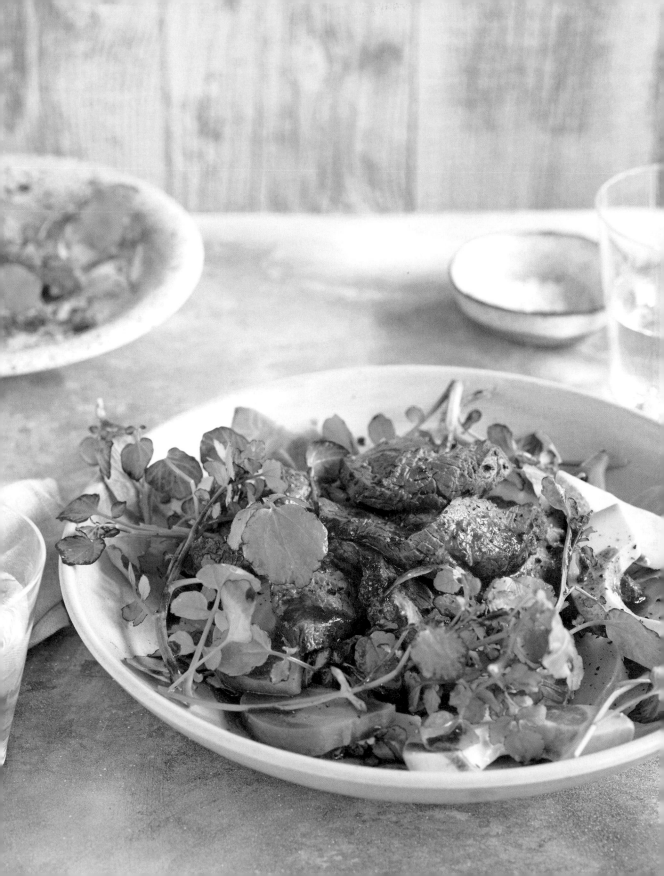

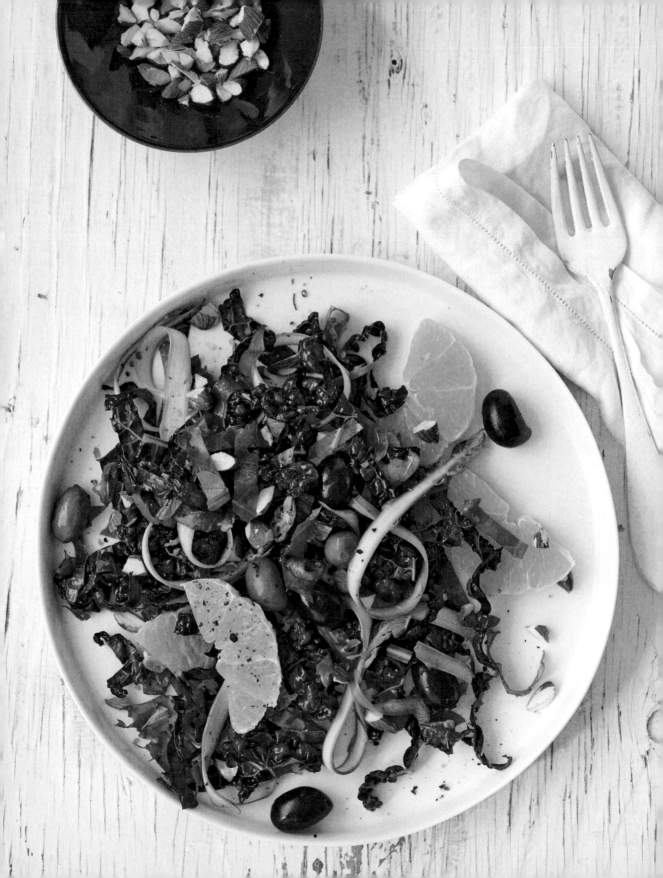

Marinated Kale Salad with Shaved Asparagus, Olives, and Orange Zest SERVES 4

Marinating kale softens its texture, which helps if you find kale chewy or tough. Unlike other salad greens, dressed kale can be stored for up to three days in the fridge, making it a great leftover for a fast lunch or healthy afternoon snack.

One 10-ounce bunch kale, blue dwarf, curly, or lacinato, stems trimmed
1 tablespoon extra-virgin olive oil

2 oranges
1 pound asparagus, trimmed
½ cup assorted olives, pitted and chopped

½ teaspoon hot or mild paprika
½ cup sliced almonds

Tear the kale leaves and place them in a large bowl along with the olive oil. Squeeze the leaves with your fingers, crushing the kale to tenderize it, for about 1 minute. Using a microplane grater, finely grate the zest of 1 of the oranges and transfer the zest to the bowl with the kale.

Shave the asparagus using a potato peeler or mandolin. Add the asparagus to the bowl with the kale along with the olives and paprika and toss well. Refrigerate the salad for at least 1 hour.

Just before serving, prepare the oranges. Using a sharp paring knife, remove the orange peel and white pith and thinly slice the oranges. Divide the salad among four plates and top with the orange slices and almonds.

NUTRITIONAL STATS PER SERVING (2½ CUPS):
205 Calories ❖ 8g Protein ❖ 23g Carbohydrates ❖ 12g Fat (1g Saturated) ❖ 0mg Cholesterol ❖ 10g Sugars ❖ 7g Fiber ❖ 157mg Sodium

Vitamin K = 699% ❖ Vitamin C = 169% ❖ Vitamin A = 86% ❖ Fiber = 28% ❖ Iron, Thiamine = 27%

Try using leftover salad in a high-fiber wrap with a tablespoon of mayo or slice of cheese, which makes for a delicious, nutrient-dense lunch.

Grilled Summer Bounty with Lemon-Herb Mayonnaise SERVES 4

Load up your grill with plants this grilling season, and then slather them in homemade mayonnaise. Made from eggs and olive oil, it's a quick and healthy addition to your veggies. The secret to the recipe is the immersion blender, which emulsifies the egg yolk perfectly without making it watery.

Mayonnaise

1 extra-large pasture-raised egg, at room temperature

1 cup light olive oil

1 teaspoon salt

½ teaspoon Dijon mustard

1 garlic clove

Finely grated zest of 1 lemon

2 tablespoons fresh lemon juice

¼ cup finely chopped fresh herbs such as basil, parsley, or tarragon

Grilled Vegetables

1 eggplant, cut into 1-inch-thick slices

4 portobello mushrooms, gills removed

2 zucchini, cut into 1-inch-thick slices

1 red bell pepper, seeded and quartered

4 tomatoes, halved

Olive oil cooking spray

2 tablespoons mixed chopped fresh herbs

½ teaspoon salt

¼ teaspoon freshly ground black pepper

Put the egg, oil, salt, mustard, and garlic in a tall narrow jar and allow the yolk to settle to the bottom. Using an immersion or stick blender, insert the blender top into the jar, making sure it stays below the oil and rests on the bottom. Blend for about 30 seconds, without lifting the blender head, until a thick pale mayonnaise forms. Blend in the lemon zest and juice and add the ¼ cup herbs last. Refrigerate in an airtight container and consume within 5 days.

Preheat a grill over high heat. Spread out the veggies on two ungreased baking sheets and coat both sides with olive oil spray. Sprinkle with the 2 tablespoons

herbs, salt, and black pepper, and transfer to the grill. Grill the veggies for 4 to 5 minutes, turning often, until soft, removing the softer vegetables such as the tomatoes first as they become charred and are cooked through. Transfer the veggies to a large platter and serve with the mayonnaise as the dipping sauce.

NUTRITIONAL STATS PER SERVING (3 CUPS VEGGIES WITH 3 TABLESPOONS MAYO): 267 Calories ❖ 6g Protein ❖ 21g Carbohydrates ❖ 19g Fat (3g Saturated) ❖ 15mg Cholesterol ❖ 12g Sugars ❖ 9g Fiber ❖ 230mg Sodium

Vitamin C = 117% ❖ Vitamin K = 53% ❖ Fiber = 38% ❖ Selenium = 35% ❖ Folate = 29%

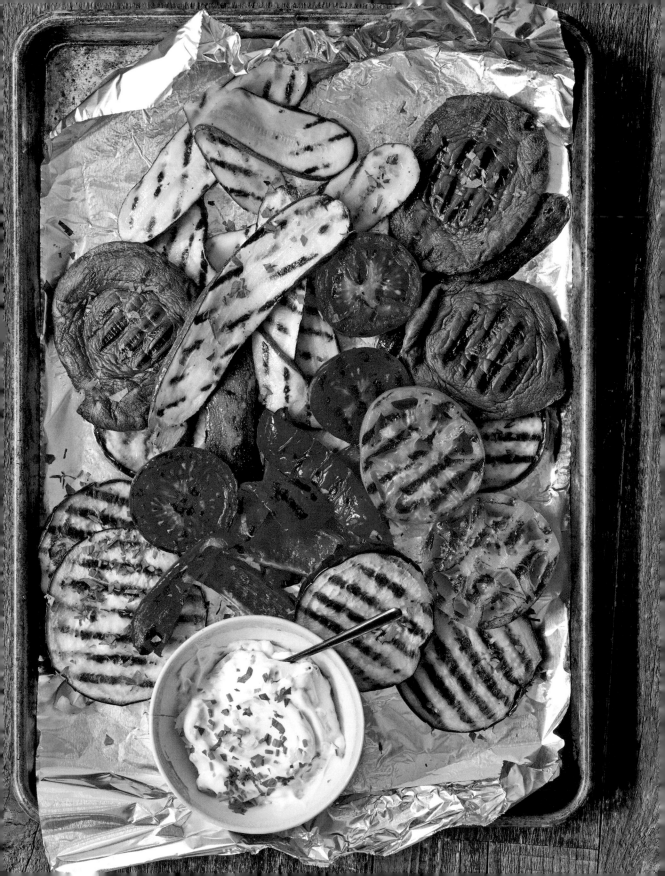

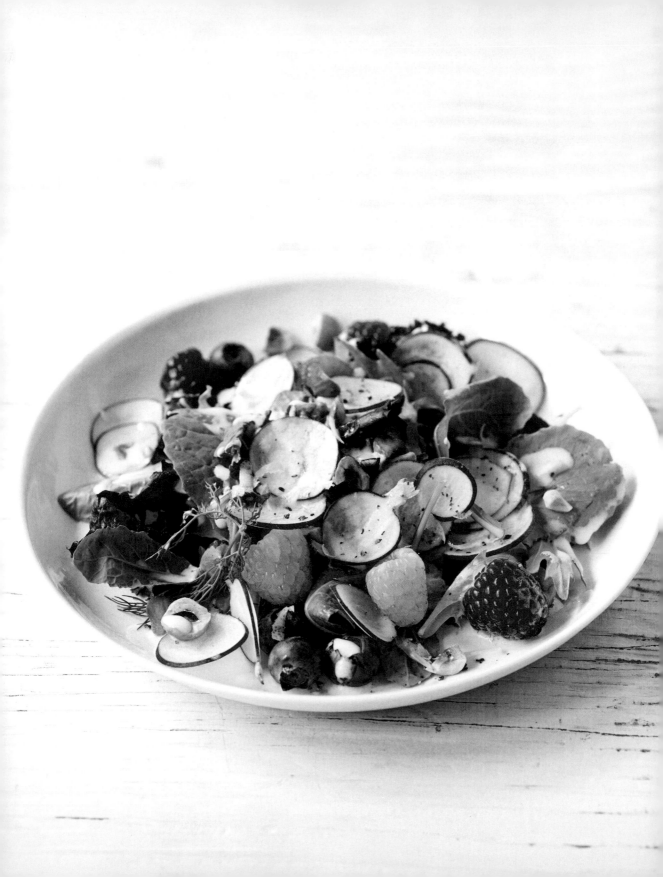

Berry Spinach Salad with Toasted Hazelnuts SERVES 4

If you love sweet and salty paired in one dish, then this nourishing salad is for you. To take this dish on the road, pack the berries and the dressing separately to avoid wilting the greens. For a cocktail party, swap the greens out for lettuce cups and spoon them full of the carrots, radishes, berries, and nuts, then drizzle with dressing.

⅓ cup hazelnuts

¼ cup extra-virgin olive oil

Juice and finely grated zest of 1 lemon

2 tablespoons plain kefir

1 teaspoon honey

½ teaspoon salt

¼ teaspoon freshly ground black pepper

½ pound salad greens, such as mesclun, baby kale, or spinach

4 carrots, peeled and thinly sliced

2 cups radishes, trimmed and thinly sliced

1 pint berries such as raspberries or blueberries

Preheat the oven or toaster oven to 350°F.

Spread out the hazelnuts in a single layer on a rimmed baking sheet. Toast in the oven until the skins split and the nuts turn a deep golden brown, 10 to 12 minutes. While still hot, rub the hazelnuts in a clean kitchen towel to remove the skins (some bits of skin will remain). Cool for 5 minutes, then chop.

Combine the oil, lemon zest and lemon juice, kefir, honey, salt, and pepper in a small bowl and whisk until smooth. Divide the salad greens among four plates. Top with the carrots, radishes, and berries and drizzle with the dressing. Garnish with the chopped hazelnuts and serve immediately.

NUTRITIONAL STATS PER SERVING (3 CUPS): 259 Calories ❖ 4g Protein ❖ 17g Carbohydrates ❖ 20g Fat (2g Saturated) ❖ 0mg Cholesterol ❖ 7g Sugars ❖ 6g Fiber ❖ 332mg Sodium

Vitamin C = 48% ❖ Vitamin A = 27% ❖ Fiber = 24% ❖ Vitamin K = 18% ❖ Magnesium = 13%

Double-Green Summer Fritters SERVES 4

Fried food doesn't have to be bad for you, and one way to keep it healthier is by frying with a healthy fat—and using less of it. Olive oil is high in monounsaturated fats (MUFAs), and eating more of these fats is linked to a lower risk of heart disease and of depression. Panfrying, rather than deep-frying, also means you can control calories while still getting things crispy! A cast-iron skillet is best for panfrying and is easy to clean (just follow the manufacturer's guide).

4 cups thinly sliced trimmed mustard greens or watercress

½ cup fresh tarragon or basil, chopped (optional)

2 pasture-raised eggs, lightly beaten

½ cup grated Parmesan cheese

¼ cup ground flaxseeds or hemp seeds

½ teaspoon baking powder

¼ teaspoon salt

3 tablespoons olive oil

¼ teaspoon freshly ground pepper

½ pound salad greens such as mesclun, baby spinach, or kale

2 tablespoons red wine vinegar or balsamic vinegar

Combine the mustard greens or watercress, the chopped tarragon or basil (if using), the eggs, Parmesan, flaxseeds or hemp seeds, baking powder, salt, and pepper in a large bowl. Stir well to coat the greens with the eggs and form a loose batter.

Coat a large skillet with 1 tablespoon olive oil and place over medium-high heat. Using a ¼-cup measure, pour out 4 mounds of batter. Cook the fritters for 2 to 3 minutes on each side until lightly browned. Mist or brush the tops with oil, then flip and cook another 2 minutes until the fritters are firm. Transfer to a plate and keep warm. Repeat making fritters with the remaining batter.

Toss the salad greens in a bowl with the remaining olive oil and vinegar. Divide the salad greens equally among four plates and top with two fritters each. Serve immediately.

NUTRITIONAL STATS PER SERVING (2 FRITTERS AND 2 CUPS SALAD GREENS): 208 Calories ❖ 11g Protein ❖ 8g Carbohydrates ❖ 15g Fat (4g Saturated) ❖ 102mg Cholestero ❖ 2g Sugars ❖ 5g Fiber ❖ 410mg Sodium

Vitamin K = 523% ❖ ALA = 157% ❖ Vitamin C = 72% ❖ Vitamin A = 61% ❖ Folate = 47%

Beet Greens with Homemade Citrus Wild Salmon Gravlax MAKES 2 POUNDS (16 SERVINGS)

Homemade gravlax is made with a simple salt and sugar cure. Use wild salmon for more brain-building, mood-boosting, long-chained omega-3 fats. Beets are a "twofer" vegetable, with both greens and roots offering potassium; vitamins A, C, and K; and phytonutrients. Buy a pound of beets for the greens, and use the beets for the Grilled Grass-Fed Beef and Watercress Salad, page 174.

⅔ cup kosher salt
⅓ cup sugar
2 tablespoons finely grated citrus zest

One 2-pound skin-on wild salmon fillet
½ pound beet greens
2 tablespoons olive oil

2 tablespoons red wine vinegar or apple cider vinegar
2 lemons or limes, cut into wedges, for garnish

In a large bowl, combine the salt, sugar, and citrus zest. Spread out one large piece of plastic wrap; sprinkle with half the salt mixture. Place the salmon fillet on top, skin side down, and cover with the remaining salt mixture. Make sure the entire fillet is covered with the salt mixture.

Fold the plastic wrap around the salmon, then wrap tightly with more plastic wrap. Place the fish in a shallow dish or platter and refrigerate for 48 to 72 hours, flipping the packet every 12 hours. When fully cured, the gravlax will be firmer to the touch and a shade darker.

Unwrap the salmon. Rinse the fillet under cold running water and pat dry with paper towels.

Before serving, place gravlax, skin side down, on a cutting board. With a long, sharp, narrow-bladed knife, slice the gravlax against the grain, on the diagonal, into thin pieces.

Toss the greens in a large bowl along with the olive oil and vinegar. Divide the greens equally among four plates and top each with a few slices of the gravlax. Serve with lemon or lime wedges. Refrigerate any remaining gravlax, well wrapped in plastic wrap, and consume within 2 weeks.

NUTRITIONAL STATS PER SERVING (⅛ POUND GRAVLAX AND 2 CUPS GREENS): 326 Calories ❖ 24g Protein ❖ 8g Carbohydrates ❖ 24g Fat (5g Saturated) ❖ 61mg Cholesterol ❖ 1g Sugars ❖ 4g Fiber ❖ 464mg Sodium

Vitamin K = 166% ❖ Vitamin C = 69% ❖ Protein = 52% ❖ Iodine = 43% ❖ Choline = 31%

183

Charbroiled Cauliflower Steak over Teff Risotto SERVES 4

Creamy teff makes a luscious base for charbroiled cauliflower that's been crisped under the broiler. Peppadew, a pepper from South Africa, is a cultivar that you can find increasingly more frequently in US grocery stores. The small peppers are convenient to use, and add a burst of sweet spiciness here that lifts the mellow flavors of the teff and cauliflower.

1 head cauliflower
2 tablespoons coconut oil
One 5-ounce container fresh mushrooms, any variety, thinly sliced
½ red onion, thinly sliced

4 scallions, green and white parts, thinly sliced
½ cup teff
1½ cups water
½ cup grated Parmesan cheese

½ teaspoon salt
¼ teaspoon freshly ground black pepper
½ teaspoon paprika
¼ cup peppadew peppers, thinly sliced

Remove the green outer leaves from the cauliflower. To form the "steak," cut a thick slice about 2 inches wide from the center of the cauliflower, cutting from top to bottom and leaving the stem intact. Reserve the remaining cauliflower for another recipe such as cauliflower hash (see page 225)

Prepare the risotto. Heat a large saucepan over medium heat, and put in 1 tablespoon of the coconut oil. Add the mushrooms, red onion, and scallions and cook for 4 to 5 minutes until the mushrooms and onions soften. Add the teff and the water and bring to a boil over high heat. Reduce the heat to low, cover, and cook for 12 to 15 minutes until most of the water has evaporated and the teff is creamy and tender to the bite. Remove from the heat, and stir in the Parmesan.

While the teff is cooking, heat a large skillet with the remaining 1 tablespoon coconut oil over medium heat, and add the cauliflower steak. Reduce the heat to low, cover, and allow the cauliflower to brown for 10 minutes. Turn the cauliflower steak and season with the salt, pepper, and paprika. Cover and cook until tender, about 10 minutes more.

Spoon the teff mixture onto a platter, and top with the cauliflower steak. Sprinkle with the peppadews and serve immediately.

NUTRITIONAL STATS PER SERVING: 225 Calories ❖ 10g Protein ❖ 24g Carbohydrates ❖ 10g Fat (3g Saturated) ❖ 9mg Cholesterol ❖ 2g Sugars ❖ 4g Fiber ❖ 470mg Sodium

Vitamin C = 43% ❖ Vitamin K = 42% ❖ Protein = 22% ❖ Zinc = 20% ❖ Magnesium, Calcium = 18%

Warm Dandelion Greens with Farmhouse Cheese and Toasted Pine Nuts SERVES 4

Bitter dandelion greens are mellowed with rich cheese and crunchy pine nuts. Look for dandelion leaves in the spring.

1 tablespoon sesame oil or pumpkin oil
1 tablespoon chopped lemon zest

2 garlic cloves, thinly sliced
½ pound dandelion greens
1 tablespoon tamari or balsamic vinegar

½ pound baby spinach
4 ounces farmhouse cheese or feta, crumbled
¼ cup pine nuts, toasted

Warm the oil in a cast-iron skillet or another large skillet over medium heat. Add the lemon zest and garlic and cook for 2 to 3 minutes, stirring often, until the garlic becomes fragrant. Add the dandelion greens, toss to coat, and cook for about 1 minute more. Turn off the heat and add the tamari or balsamic vinegar and toss to coat.

Divide the spinach among four plates and top with the wilted dandelions and cheese. Sprinkle with the toasted pine nuts and serve immediately.

NUTRITIONAL STATS PER SERVING (2 CUPS): 193 Calories ❖ 7g Protein ❖ 8g Carbohydrates ❖ 15g Fat (5g Saturated) ❖ 25mg Cholesterol ❖ 2g Sugars ❖ 2g Fiber ❖ 530mg Sodium

Vitamin K = 496% ❖ Vitamin A = 46% ❖ Thiamine = 36% ❖ Vitamin C = 29% ❖ Calcium = 25%

Deconstructed Lobster Roll Salad with Creamy Old Bay Dressing SERVES 4

Liberate lobster from the hot dog bun! Lobster rolls are tempting fare, but white bread rolls and the accompanying french fries turn them into junk food. This deconstructed version keeps a lot of the goodness while bringing a fresh healthy makeover, by pulling out the lobster, creamy dressing, and crunchy celery and combining them with fresh greens instead of empty carbohydrates.

¼ cup buttermilk, preferably from grass-fed cows

¼ cup olive oil–based mayonnaise

¼ cup chopped fresh flat-leaf parsley

2 scallions, minced

1 teaspoon reduced-sodium Old Bay seasoning

¼ teaspoon freshly ground black pepper

1 pound baby greens, such as romaine, beet greens, kale, or spinach

4 cooked lobster tails, shelled and meat chopped

4 celery stalks, finely diced

1 cup fresh corn kernels or defrosted frozen corn kernels

Prepare the dressing. Place the buttermilk, mayonnaise, parsley, scallions, Old Bay seasoning, and pepper in a blender and process. Set aside.

Arrange the baby greens, distributing them equally, on four plates. Top with the lobster meat, celery, and corn, dividing them equally. Drizzle the dressing over the salad and serve immediately.

NUTRITIONAL STATS PER SERVING (MEAT FROM 1 LOBSTER TAIL AND 3 CUPS SALAD): 215 Calories ❖ 24g Protein ❖ 14g Carbohydrates ❖ 6g Fat (0g Saturated) ❖ 112mg Cholesterol ❖ 4g Sugars ❖ 3g Fiber ❖ 595mg Sodium

Vitamin K = 212% ❖ Selenium = 87% ❖ Vitamin A = 78% ❖ Folate, Protein = 52% ❖ Zinc = 49%

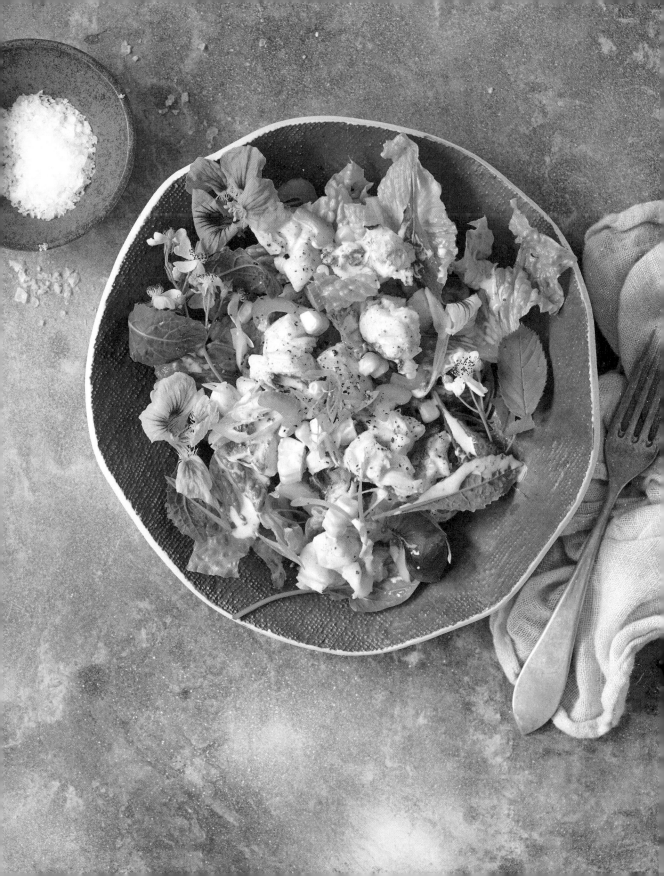

Black Bean Salad with Toasted Cumin Seeds SERVES 4

This summery salad calls on the phytonutrient power of black beans, an unsung hero of the superfood world. In addition to providing ample protein, fiber, and B vitamins, beans top the charts of antioxidant power. To keep sodium in check, your best bet is to shop for low-sodium canned bean varieties in health food stores, as the brands they carry tend to be 25 to 50 percent lower in salt compared with "lower sodium" options in traditional grocery stores. Look for BPA-free cans to avoid this toxin. You can also soak dried organic beans overnight for the best value.

⅓ cup fresh lime juice

2 tablespoons extra-virgin olive oil

2 teaspoons mild chili powder

¼ teaspoon salt

¼ teaspoon ground cayenne pepper (or mild chili powder)

2 teaspoons cumin seeds

Two 15-ounce cans low-sodium black beans, rinsed well under cold running water and drained

3 ears fresh corn, kernels cut off the cob (about 3 cups)

2 red bell peppers, seeded and diced

½ cup chopped fresh cilantro, plus more for garnish

2 tablespoons minced red onion or shallot

2 garlic cloves, minced

2 Hass avocados

Put the lime juice, olive oil, chili powder, salt, and cayenne in a large bowl and whisk to combine. Set the dressing aside.

Place a small dry skillet over medium heat. Put in the cumin seeds and toast until fragrant. Transfer to the bowl with the dressing and add the beans, corn, bell peppers, cilantro, red onion or shallot, and garlic. Toss well to coat. Cover the salad and chill for a few hours or overnight.

Just before serving, pit, peel, and chop the avocados and toss gently with the salad. Serve cold or at room temperature.

NUTRITIONAL STATS PER SERVING (2 CUPS): 485 Calories ❖ 17g Protein ❖ 67g Carbohydrates ❖ 20g Fat (2g Saturated) ❖ 0mg Cholesterol ❖ 7g Sugars ❖ 19g Fiber ❖ 208mg Sodium

Vitamin C = 124% ❖ Fiber = 78% ❖ Protein = 38% ❖ Vitamin A = 36% ❖ Vitamin K, Folate = 33%

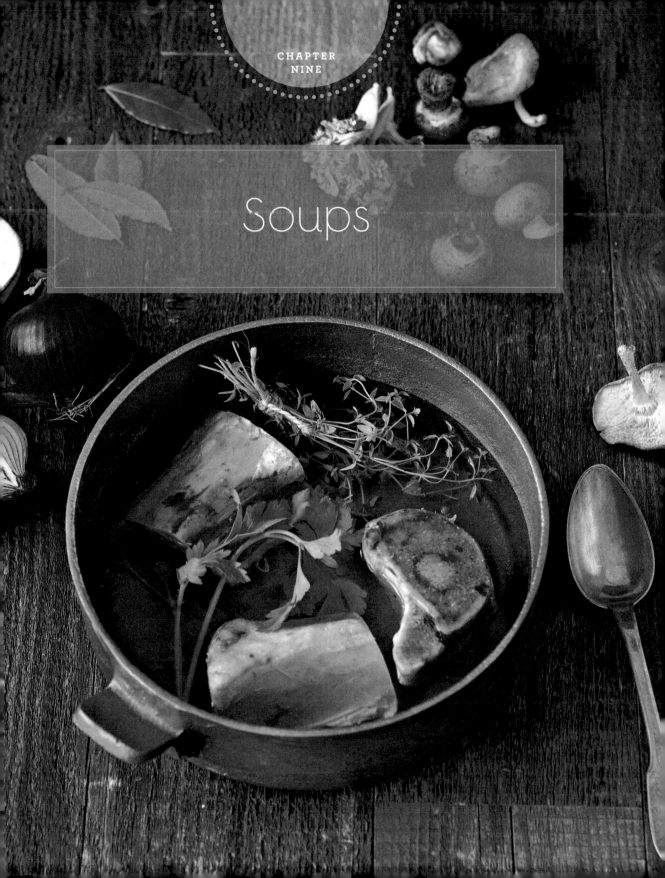

Soups

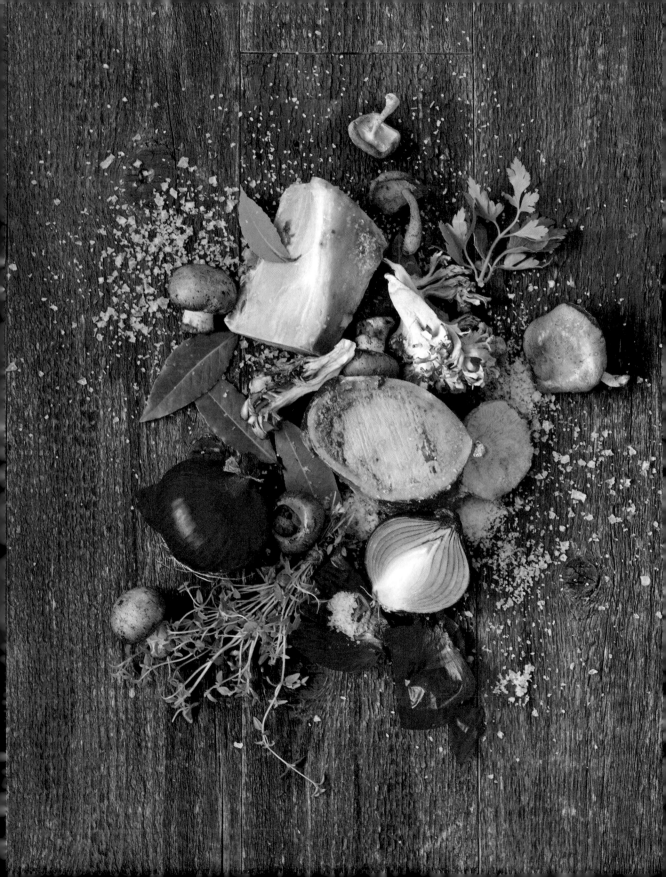

Pumpkin Soup with Cinnamon Macadamia Nuts SERVES 4

Pumpkins get their color from the high concentration of carotenoids (see page 60). For a fast and easy version, canned organic pumpkin is nutritionally equivalent to fresh. Cinnamon is a top spice for antioxidant power.

1 small pumpkin, about 2 pounds, peeled and cubed, or two 15.5-ounce cans 100 percent pure organic pumpkin

1 tablespoon olive oil

1 red or white onion, chopped

½ teaspoon freshly ground black pepper

6 cups bone broth (see page 200) or low-sodium chicken broth

½ cup macadamia nuts

⅓ cup sunflower seeds

¼ teaspoon ground cinnamon

1 tablespoon honey

1 tablespoon water

1 teaspoon pure vanilla extract

Preheat the oven to 400°F. Peel and cube the pumpkin. If using fresh pumpkin, put half of the olive oil in a large stockpot over medium heat. Add the pumpkin cubes, onion, and pepper and cover. Reduce the heat to low and cook for 3 to 4 minutes, stirring occasionally, until the pumpkin begins to brown. Add the broth and cover. Cook for 4 to 5 minutes more until the pumpkin is tender. Using an immersion blender, blend the pumpkin until smooth.

If using the canned pumpkin, put half of the oil in a large stockpot and warm over medium heat. Add the onion and cook for 3 to 4 minutes, stirring often, until the onion starts to brown. Add the canned pumpkin and the broth, and cook for 3 to 4 minutes more, stirring well. Using an immersion blender, blend until smooth.

Warm the remaining oil in a medium ovenproof skillet over medium heat. Add the macadamia nuts, sunflower seeds, and cinnamon and stir to coat. Add the honey, water, and vanilla extract. Transfer the skillet to the oven and bake the nut-seed mixture for 5 to 6 minutes, stirring occasionally, until golden. Remove from the oven and cool for 2 minutes.

Spoon the soup into bowls and sprinkle with the nut mixture. Serve immediately.

NUTRITIONAL STATS PER SERVING (½ CUP): 308
Calories ❖ 11g Protein ❖ 28g Carbohydrates ❖ 18g Fat (3g Saturated) ❖ 7mg Cholesterol ❖ 11g Sugars ❖ 4g Fiber ❖ 255mg Sodium

Vitamin A = 120% ❖ Vitamin C = 29% ❖ Thiamine = 27% ❖ Protein = 26% ❖ Magnesium and Selenium = 20%

Pumpkin Soup with Cinnamon
Macadamia Nuts; Heirloom
Tomato Gazpacho

Heirloom Tomato Gazpacho SERVES 4

The world of tomato varietals is vast—from black to pink, five pounders to pearls—and heirlooms are prized for their flavor and survival abilities. Watercress and hemp seeds add a boost to this traditional Spanish cold soup, which is a simple salute to fruits and vegetables. No cooking means a total preservation of the heat-sensitive nutrients such as vitamin C and folate, which are found in both the tomatoes and the peppers. The olive oil is essential to boost your absorption of the many fat-soluble phytonutrients in the tomatoes, such as lycopene. To make this a more filling meal, top each serving with 4 ounces of grilled shrimp, scallops, or chicken.

2 pounds heirloom tomatoes, quartered

1 red bell pepper, seeded and chopped

2 cups watercress

½ cup chopped red onion

¼ cup hemp seeds

2 tablespoons sherry vinegar

1 tablespoon extra-virgin olive oil

1 tablespoon fresh lemon juice

½ teaspoon salt

¼ cup chopped fresh cilantro leaves or microgreens

Place the tomatoes, pepper, watercress, red onion, hemp seeds, vinegar, oil, lemon juice, and salt in a blender or food processor and blend until smooth. Serve immediately, or refrigerate up to 1 day before serving. Sprinkle with the chopped cilantro or microgreens just before serving.

NUTRITIONAL STATS PER SERVING (2 CUPS): 143
Calories ❖ 5g Protein ❖ 15g Carbohydrates ❖
9g Fat (1g Saturated) ❖ 0mg Cholesterol ❖
8g Sugars ❖ 5g Fiber ❖ 306mg Sodium

Vitamin C = 87% ❖ Vitamin K = 76% ❖
Magnesium = 39% ❖ Thiamine = 27% ❖ Zinc = 25%

If you can't find heirloom tomatoes, or if you hanker for this soup out of season, you can use beefsteak tomatoes instead.

French Onion-Leek Soup SERVES 4

When the traditional indulgence of French onion soup meets white beans, the results are nutritionally astounding and surprisingly filling. Yes, this still includes onions, rich broth, and cheese, but one serving delivers at least half of your daily need for five key nutrients—folate, vitamin K, vitamin A, fiber, and vitamin C—plus a third of your daily iron. This hunger-busting soup can double as a satisfying meal instead of just a first course, as the protein, fiber, and fats in the beans, onions, and cheese keep you feeling fuller, longer. The seasonal option of garlic scapes is a must-try on a cold, rainy spring day.

1 tablespoon extra-virgin olive oil

2 large sweet onions, peeled and sliced

4 leeks, white and light green parts, chopped

1 teaspoon chopped fresh thyme

½ teaspoon salt

¼ teaspoon freshly ground pepper

4 cups bone broth (see page 200) or two 15.5-ounce cans no-salt-added beef broth

One 15.5-ounce can navy beans, rinsed well under

cold running water and drained

1 tablespoon sherry vinegar or apple cider vinegar

¼ cup minced fresh chives or garlic scapes

½ cup shredded grass-fed Gruyère or Swiss cheese, or 4 thin slices

Heat the oil in a large saucepan over medium-high heat. Add the onions and leeks and stir to coat with the oil. Cover; reduce the heat to medium; and cook, stirring often, until the onions are soft and starting to brown, 6 to 8 minutes. Add the thyme, salt, and pepper. Reduce the heat to low and cook, uncovered, stirring often, until the onions become a deep golden brown, 20 to 25 minutes. If the onions and leeks begin to stick or threaten to burn, add a tablespoon of water.

Stir in the broth, navy beans, and sherry vinegar or apple cider vinegar and bring to a simmer over high heat. Cook for 1 minute

to allow the flavors to meld. Turn off the heat and stir in the chives or garlic scapes.

Ladle the soup into four large oven-safe bowls and top with cheese. Place under the broiler for 1 minute until the cheese has melted. Serve immediately.

NUTRITIONAL STATS PER SERVING (2 CUPS): 371 Calories ❖ 20g Protein ❖ 44g Carbohydrates ❖ 12g Fat (5g Saturated) ❖ 18mg Cholesterol ❖ 7g Sugars ❖ 13g Fiber ❖ 750mg Sodium

Vitamin K = 200% ❖ Vitamin A = 100% ❖ Folate = 54% ❖ Fiber = 52% ❖ Vitamin C = 49%

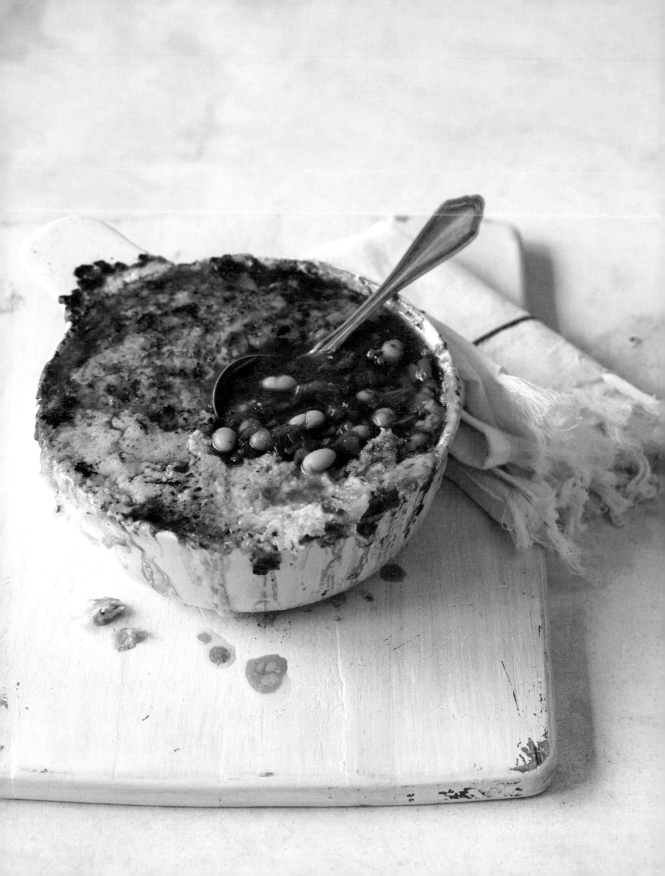

Chilled Avocado-Cucumber-Dill Soup SERVES 4

Looking for a no-cook, brain-boosting option for lunch or dinner? Soothe your overworked brain with this inflammation-cooling blend of plants. Avocados are a unique fruit given their high content of monounsaturated fats, which help you absorb the fat-soluble nutrients from the eight other plant ingredients. Make this meal in minutes for fresh-tasting satisfaction. Cilantro will substitute nicely if you don't have basil on hand. You can also make this more of a meal by adding protein, such as a dollop of sour cream or Greek yogurt.

2 Hass avocados, pitted and peeled

2 cups low-sodium chicken or vegetable broth

1 green apple, cored and chopped

1 large cucumber, peeled and chopped

¼ cup chopped fresh dill

2 celery stalks, chopped

¼ cup sherry vinegar or apple cider vinegar

2 tablespoons extra-virgin olive oil, plus more for drizzling

1 garlic clove, peeled and halved

¼ teaspoon salt

4 sprigs fresh basil

Place the avocados, broth, apple, cucumber, dill, celery, vinegar, olive oil, garlic, and salt in a blender or food processor and blend until smooth. Transfer the soup to the fridge and chill at least 1 hour before serving.

Spoon the chilled soup into four bowls and top with the basil.

NUTRITIONAL STATS PER SERVING (2 CUPS): 254
Calories ❖ 5g Protein ❖ 19g Carbohydrates ❖ 18g Fat (2g Saturated) ❖ 2mg Cholesterol ❖ 8g Sugars ❖ 6g Fiber ❖ 340mg Sodium

Vitamin K = 42% ❖ Fiber = 26% ❖ Folate = 20% ❖ Vitamin C = 16% ❖ Potassium = 14%

Chicken-on-the-Bone Soup with Sofrito SERVES 4

Cooking chicken on the bone ensures this delicate meat doesn't dry out. A savory mixture of onions, garlic, peppers, and cilantro gives this soup a Latin flair, and sets it apart from run-of-the-mill chicken soup. Noodles are swapped out here for amaranth, a gluten-free grain with high amounts of protein, iron, and magnesium—nutrients you need to build the molecules in your brain that create a smile.

2 bone-in, skin-on chicken breasts

¼ teaspoon freshly ground black pepper

1 tablespoon olive oil

1 red or yellow onion, peeled and diced

4 carrots, peeled and chopped

4 parsnips, peeled and chopped

2 jalapeños or green bell peppers, seeded and chopped

½ cup packed fresh cilantro, chopped

2 garlic cloves, minced

1 quart low-sodium chicken broth

¼ cup amaranth

Sprinkle the chicken with the black pepper.

Heat the olive oil in a large stockpot over medium heat. Add the chicken breasts, skin side down, and cook for 1 to 2 minutes until the skins start to brown and give off some of their fat. Remove the chicken breasts from the pot and place on a plate.

Add the onion, carrots, parsnips, jalapeños or green peppers, cilantro, and garlic to the pot and cook for 3 to 4 minutes until the vegetables start to soften.

Add the broth and amaranth and bring to a boil over high heat. Reduce to a simmer and cook for 10 minutes.

Return the chicken to the broth and cook for 10 minutes more. Turn off the heat, cover, and set aside for 20 minutes until the chicken is cooked through and no longer pink at the bone.

Transfer the chicken to a cutting board and let cool slightly, 5 to 6 minutes. Remove and discard the skin and shred the meat. Return the meat to the soup along with the vegetables. Serve immediately.

NUTRITIONAL STATS PER SERVING (2 CUPS): 368 Calories ❖ 27g Protein ❖ 39g Carbohydrates ❖ 11g Fat (2g Saturated) ❖ 82mg Cholesterol ❖ 12g Sugars ❖ 8g Fiber ❖ 584mg Sodium

Vitamin A = 148% ❖ Vitamin C = 73% ❖ Protein = 59% ❖ Selenium = 56% ❖ Vitamin K = 48%

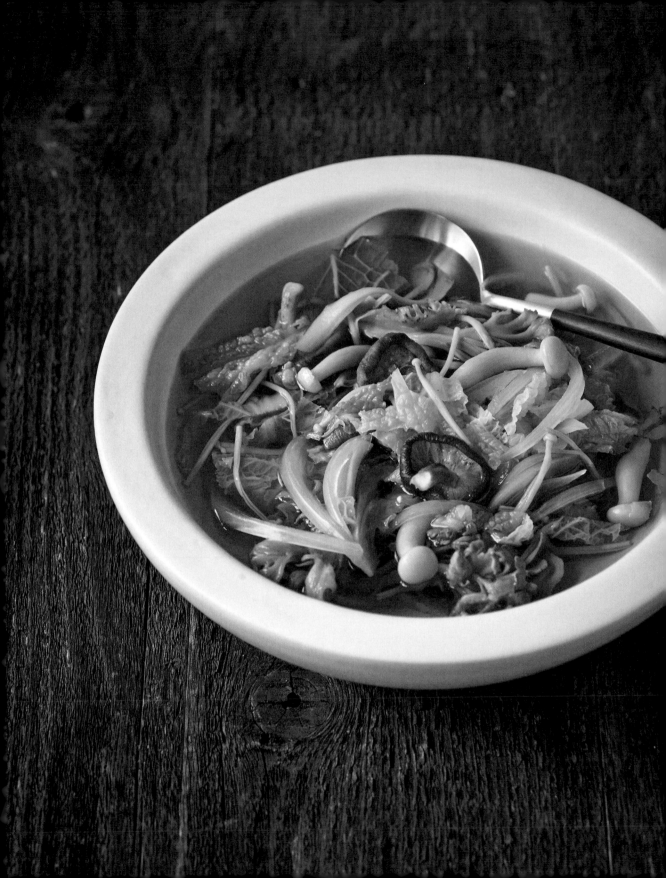

Green Tea Mushroom Soup SERVES 4

Can you imagine a cup of soup for lunch that is both therapeutic and caffeinated? Tea and soup are two healing liquids that work well together in this flavorful Asian-inspired recipe. A variety of antioxidants from both the plant and the fungus phytonutrients are infused into every sip, helping you fight inflammation, aging, and fatigue. If you're sensitive to caffeine, opt for decaffeinated tea. Leftover collards or kale can be swapped in for the cabbage.

1 tablespoon sesame oil
½ pound mushrooms such as oyster, shiitake, or hen-of-the-woods
1 red or yellow onion, minced
2 garlic cloves, minced

6 cups low-sodium chicken broth, bone broth (see page 200), or vegetable broth
4 cups thinly sliced Napa cabbage

2 green tea bags
1 tablespoon low-sodium tamari or 2 teaspoons Bragg's Liquid Aminos (optional)
¼ cup sesame seeds

Heat the sesame oil in a large stockpot over medium heat. Add the mushrooms, onion, and garlic and cook for 4 to 5 minutes until the mushrooms soften. Add the broth, bring to a boil over high heat, and immediately reduce to a simmer. Add the cabbage and cook for 4 to 5 minutes until tender.

Turn off the heat, add the green tea bags, and let steep for 3 minutes. Remove and discard the tea bags.

Stir in the tamari or Bragg's Liquid Aminos, if using. Serve immediately, sprinkled with the sesame seeds.

NUTRITIONAL STATS PER SERVING (2 CUPS): 258 Calories ❖ 14g Protein ❖ 24g Carbohydrates ❖ 12g Fat (2g Saturated) ❖ 10mg Cholesterol ❖ 8g Sugars ❖ 3g Fiber ❖ 404mg Sodium

Vitamin K = 38% ❖ Vitamin C = 31% ❖ Protein = 30% ❖ Folate = 29% ❖ Thiamine = 27%

Bone Broth with Torn Greens SERVES 4

Stewing bones yields original broth. Rich in amino acids and flavor, broths can be very soothing and therapeutic for the gut due to high amounts of the amino acid glycine—and your gut must be healthy to absorb all the nutrients required by your brain. Use the extra broth for several of the other recipes. Adding greens and grains adds more nutrients and turns a simple broth into a more complete meal supercharged with minerals, vitamins, and phytonutrients.

1 tablespoon safflower or olive oil

3 pounds beef marrow and knucklebones

2 pounds beef shank bones or oxtails or meaty bones such as short ribs

2 tablespoons tomato paste

½ cup raw apple cider vinegar

3 quarts water

3 celery stalks, halved

3 carrots, halved

3 onions, quartered

½ cup fresh flat-leaf parsley stems and leaves

Pinch of salt

¼ cup uncooked amaranth or teff

4 cups packed collard or kale leaves, torn

Warm the oil in a large stockpot over medium-high heat. Add the bones in batches and cook for 4 to 5 minutes, turning often, until they are browned. When you brown the last batch, add the tomato paste. Return all the bones to the stockpot and add the apple cider vinegar and water.

Add the celery, carrots, onions, parsley, and salt and bring to a boil over high heat. Reduce to a low simmer, cover, and cook for 12 to 24 hours.

Let the broth cool and strain it, making sure all the marrow is knocked out of the marrow bones and into the broth.

NOTE: Store extra broth by freezing it in a jar, leaving room for expansion when it freezes. You can also freeze it in an ice cube tray, which provides convenient portions of broth whenever you need to boost the flavor and nutrient density of beans, soups, or grains.

After you strain the broth, return approximately half of it to a pot and place over medium heat. Add the amaranth or teff and cook until the grains are tender, 15 to 20 minutes. During the final 3 to 4 minutes of cooking, mix in the greens.

Serve the soup immediately or cool completely before storing in an airtight container, refrigerated for up to a week.

NUTRITIONAL STATS PER SERVING (2 CUPS): 170 Calories ❖ 11g Protein ❖ 9g Carbohydrates ❖ 3g Fat ❖ (3g Saturated) ❖ 0mg Cholesterol ❖ 2g Sugars ❖ 2g Fiber ❖ 256mg Sodium

Vitamin K = 52% ❖ Vitamin C = 48% ❖ Protein = 26% ❖ Vitamin A = 25% ❖ Iron = 14%

Spicy Shredded Beef Soup with Turnips SERVES 6

Earthy turnips and slow-cooked beef provide a brothy bowl of comfort. High amounts of zinc and vitamin C keep your immune defenses strong. Reheat leftovers on a rainy workday to soothe your stress, or store in an airtight container in the freezer for an easy winter meal to feed the family. When preparing for kids, hold the cayenne and swap in jarred salsa for the kimchee. Before you discard the turnip greens, consider sautéing them to create an easy, nutritious side. And swap water for beef stock for a richer soup.

One 2-pound piece grass-fed flank steak
1 medium onion, peeled and chopped
2 carrots, peeled and chopped
3 celery stalks, chopped
2 bay leaves
1 teaspoon whole black peppercorns
4 quarts low-sodium beef stock (optional)
1 tablespoon olive oil
1 bunch scallions, trimmed and thinly sliced on the diagonal
2 garlic cloves, minced
¼ teaspoon ground cayenne pepper (optional)
2 turnips, peeled and thinly sliced
¼ cup tomato paste
1 teaspoon salt
¼ cup prepared kimchee (optional)

In a 6-quart stockpot, place the flank steak, onion, carrots, celery, bay leaves, and peppercorns. Cover with 4 quarts of cold water or beef stock, leaving a 1-inch space from the top of the stockpot. Bring to a simmer and cook, partially covered, for 1½ to 2 hours until the beef shreds easily when pressed with a fork.

When the meat is very tender, turn off the heat and let the meat cool in the liquid for 20 minutes, before removing from the broth. Strain the broth into a large bowl and discard the vegetables. Shred the beef.

Heat the oil over medium heat in the same stockpot in which you cooked the beef.

Add the scallions, garlic, and cayenne, if using. Cook for 2 to 3 minutes until the scallions begin to soften. Add the shredded beef, broth, turnips, tomato paste, and salt and cook for 4 to 5 minutes more until the turnips soften. Garnish with kimchee, if using, and serve immediately.

NUTRITIONAL STATS PER SERVING (2 CUPS WITHOUT KIMCHEE): 359 Calories ❖ 35g Protein ❖ 20g Carbohydrates ❖ 14g Fat (5g Saturated) ❖ 70mg Cholesterol ❖ 4g Sugars ❖ 5g Fiber ❖ 524mg Sodium

Vitamin B$_{12}$ = 158% ❖ Vitamin C = 123% ❖ Zinc = 121% ❖ Selenium = 93% ❖ Protein = 76%

Creamy Caraway Carrot Soup with Fried Sage SERVES 4

Fall flavors team up in this savory soup. Beets add a layer of earthiness to the carrots and extra carotenoids, the yellow-orange pigments found in both the golden beets and the carrots. The beets also bring betaine to your table, a B vitamin–like nutrient that helps reduce markers of inflammation. And they contain natural nitrates that relax blood vessels and improve blood flow.

Frying the sage mellows it and turns the velvety leaves into crisp chips, though any fresh herb will work well instead, from basil to cilantro to parsley—no frying required. Remember that the beet greens are incredibly nutrient dense. Use them later in a salad, sauté as a side dish, or add to your smoothie.

2 tablespoons coconut oil, plus 2 teaspoons for frying the sage
6 carrots, peeled and chopped

2 large golden beets, peeled and chopped
1 onion, peeled and chopped
1 tablespoon caraway seeds
½ teaspoon ground turmeric

32 ounces low-sodium chicken broth, bone broth (see page 200), or vegetable broth
4 large fresh sage leaves

Heat a large stockpot over medium heat and put in the 2 tablespoons oil. Add the carrots, beets, onion, caraway seeds, and turmeric. Cover and cook for 4 to 5 minutes, stirring occasionally, until the carrots and beets start to brown. Add the broth, increase the heat to high, and bring to a boil. Cover, reduce immediately to a simmer, and cook for 4 to 5 minutes more until the carrots are tender. Let the soup cool for 5 minutes, then blend until smooth.

Put the remaining 2 teaspoons oil in a small skillet over medium heat. Add the sage and fry for 1 minute. Drain on a paper towel.

Divide the soup among four bowls, sprinkle with the fried sage, and serve immediately.

NUTRITIONAL STATS PER SERVING (2 CUPS): 244 Calories ❖ 8g Protein ❖ 26g Carbohydrates ❖ 12g Fat (8g Saturated) ❖ 7mg Cholesterol ❖ 12g Sugars ❖ 5g Fiber ❖ 393mg Sodium

Vitamin A = 110% ❖ Vitamin K = 24% ❖ Fiber, Vitamin C = 20% ❖ Thiamine = 18% ❖ Potassium, Protein = 17%

Curried Cauliflower–Garlic Soup with Cashews

When the scent of spice and coconut is wafting through your kitchen, no one's expecting cauliflower. Using traditional spice mixes, you can bring many of Mother Nature's most powerful compounds to the table. The curcumin in curry powder, which possesses antidementia, anticancer, antibacterial, and antidepressant properties, is a prime example. Search out curry mixes that don't contain extra sugar or salt but do contain ingredients you recognize—such as coriander, cinnamon, and especially turmeric. Garam masala is another option, an Indian spice mix that usually contains black peppercorns, mace, cardamom, and cloves; it can be located in specialty spice shops and online.

1 tablespoon coconut oil

1 head cauliflower, cut into florets (about 6 cups)

4 garlic cloves, thinly sliced

1 teaspoon curry powder or garam masala

1 quart low-sodium chicken or vegetable broth

One 15-ounce can diced tomatoes and their juices

1 cup water

2 tablespoons heavy cream

¼ cup cashews or macadamia nuts

4 scallions, thinly sliced

Warm the coconut oil in a large stockpot over medium heat. Add the cauliflower florets and cook for 6 to 8 minutes, covered, stirring occasionally, until the florets are browned and starting to soften. Add the garlic and curry powder or garam masala and cook for 1 minute more until the garlic is fragrant. Add the broth and tomatoes along with the water. Cover and cook for 4 to 5 minutes more until the cauliflower is fork-tender. Turn off the heat and blend the soup with an immersion blender. Let cool slightly and stir in the cream. Serve immediately, sprinkled with the nuts and the scallions.

NUTRITIONAL STATS PER SERVING (2 CUPS): 221
Calories ❖ 5g Protein ❖ 22g Carbohydrates ❖ 14g Fat (8g Saturated) ❖ 10mg Cholesterol ❖ 7g Sugars ❖ 5g Fiber ❖ 362mg Sodium

Vitamin C = 121% ❖ Vitamin K = 30% ❖ Folate = 23% ❖ Fiber = 20% ❖ Potassium = 17%

Summer Clam Chowder with Tomatoes, Carrots, and Shallots SERVES 4

When it comes to eating complete, don't forget the clams. Adding clams to your vegetable chowder infuses it with vitamin B_{12}, since clams are the planet's top source. This Manhattan-style-inspired chowder is also a great way to pack your veggies into a fast and flavorful meal. Shellfish is naturally high in sodium, so if you're on a sodium-restricted diet, cut the amount of clams in half to bring the sodium down.

1 pound raw clams in the shell

6 cups no-salt-added chicken broth

2 tablespoons olive oil

1 green bell pepper, seeded and diced

8 carrots, peeled and chopped

4 celery stalks, peeled and chopped

2 shallots, diced, or ½ cup diced red or yellow onion

¼ cup fresh cilantro or flat-leaf parsley, chopped

2 garlic cloves, minced

4 tomatoes, chopped

4 cups spinach, chopped

½ teaspoon crushed red pepper flakes (optional)

Rinse the clams under cold running water. Put the chicken broth in a large saucepan and bring to a boil. Add the clams and cook for 3 to 4 minutes until the clams open up. Reserve the cooking broth. Carefully remove the clamshells, roughly chop the clams, and place them in a small bowl; discard the shells.

In a large stockpot, warm the oil over medium heat. Add the bell pepper, carrots, celery, shallots or onion, cilantro or parsley, and garlic and cook for 3 to 4 minutes until the vegetables start to soften. Add the tomatoes and cook for 2 to 3 minutes more until the tomatoes give off their liquid.

Add the chicken broth you used to cook the clams, along with the spinach and red pepper flakes, if using, and bring to a simmer. Cook for 2 minutes to allow the spinach to wilt. Add the reserved clams and warm through, about 1 minute. Serve immediately.

NUTRITIONAL STATS PER SERVING (2½ CUPS):
248 Calories ❖ 13g Protein ❖ 26g Carbohydrates 10g ❖ Fat (3g Saturated) ❖ 17mg Cholesterol ❖ 12g Sugars ❖ 8g Fiber ❖ 510mg sodium

Vitamin B_{12} = 533% ❖ Vitamin K = 344% ❖ Vitamin A = 195% ❖ Selenium = 65% ❖ Vitamin C = 59%

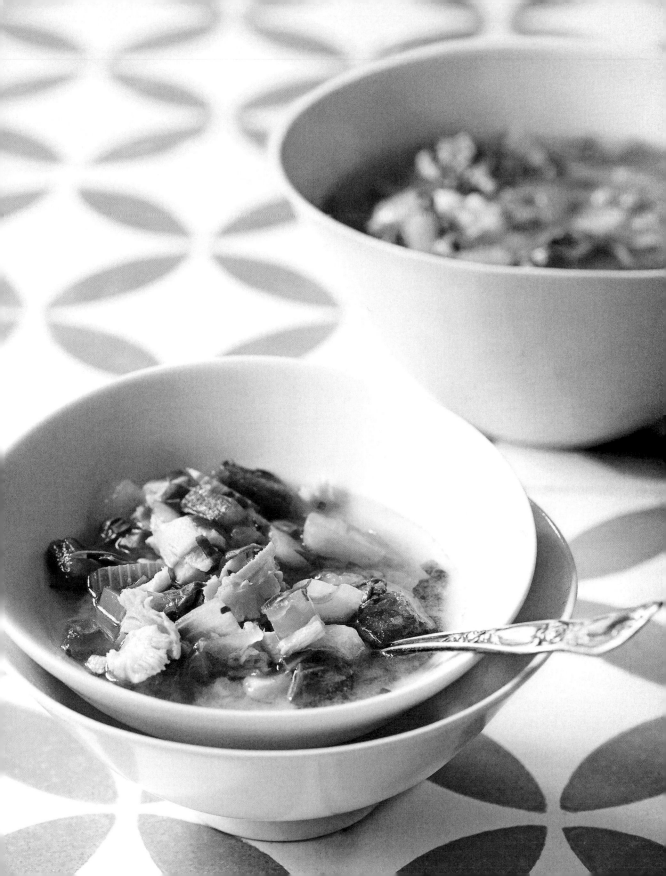

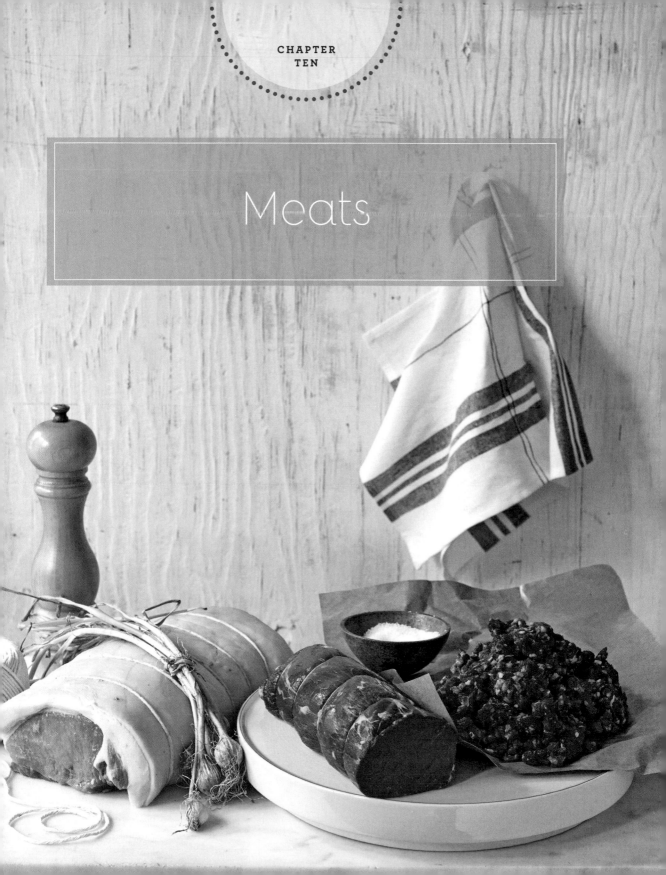

Meats

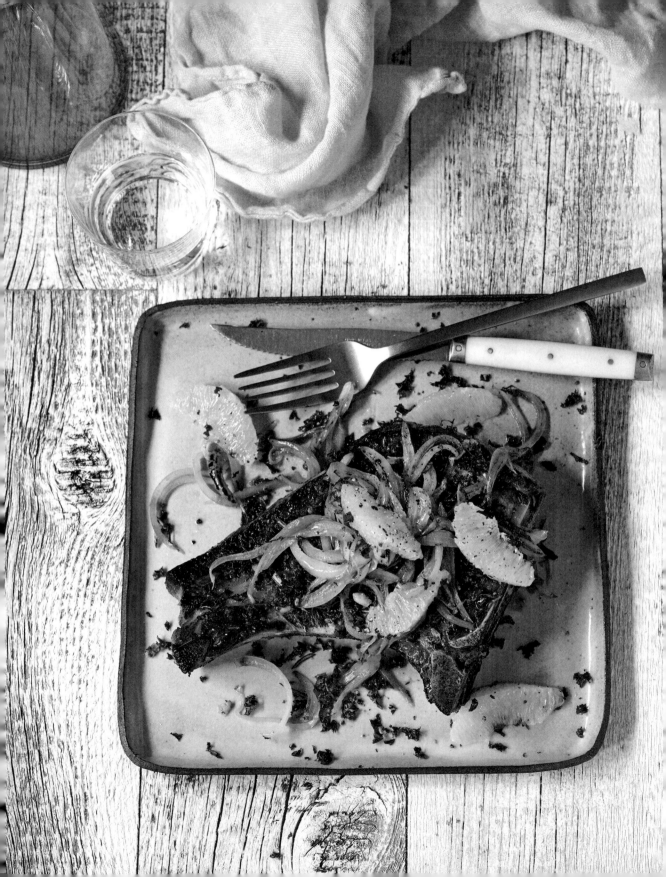

Kale-Crusted Pork Chops with Caramelized Onions and Oranges SERVES 4

This dish is superfood synergy. You've got the top source of thiamine for dinner, surrounded by all-star kale. Pork chops from an animal raised on a pasture will bring extra flavor, more nutrients, and better fats. Pork pairs well with sweet flavors like golden caramelized onions and juicy sweet oranges, plus you'll get a boost of vitamin C and phytonutrients from these and the kale. Patience is the key to caramelizing onions. Cook them slowly and lower the heat if they start to stick or burn around the edges.

4 bone-in pasture-raised pork chops

2 garlic cloves, peeled and halved

½ teaspoon salt

4 large kale leaves, stems trimmed, torn into pieces

¼ cup fresh rosemary needles

1 tablespoon fresh thyme leaves

Olive oil spray or mister

2 tablespoons olive oil

4 onions, peeled and thinly sliced

2 oranges, peeled and segmented

Preheat the oven to 400°F.

Place the pork chops on a baking sheet. Combine the garlic and ¼ teaspoon of the salt in a food processor and process until finely chopped. Add the kale, rosemary, and thyme and pulse until chunky. Spoon the kale mixture over the top of the pork chops. Spray or mist the tops of the chops with the olive oil spray and transfer to the oven. Bake for 25 to 30 minutes until the chops are no longer pink in the center and the kale coating has started to brown.

While the chops are baking prepare the onions. Warm the 2 tablespoons oil in a large skillet over medium-high heat and add the onions. Cook for 7 to 8 minutes,

stirring often, until the onions start to brown and soften. Add the remaining salt, then reduce the heat to low and continue cooking for 8 to 10 minutes until the onions are golden brown.

Transfer 1 chop to each of four plates. Top each chop with caramelized onions and the orange segments and serve.

NUTRITIONAL STATS PER SERVING (1 CHOP, ½ ORANGE, ¼ CUP ONIONS): 300 Calories ❖ 28g Protein ❖ 22g Carbohydrates ❖ 11g Fat (2g Saturated) ❖ 74mg Cholesterol ❖ 11g Sugars ❖ 4g Fiber ❖ 366mg Sodium

Vitamin K = 309% ❖ Vitamin C = 113% ❖ Thiamine = 81% ❖ Selenium = 75% ❖ Protein = 63%

Whole Roasted Chicken with Anchovies and Olives SERVES 4

Few things say "family meal" like a roasted bird. Stop in at your local Italian deli to get your provisions for this homey roasted chicken as it likely carries the best-quality brands of jarred goods. You'll appreciate the flavor that the salty anchovies and olives impart to the chicken meat when they rest under the skin during roasting. No need to truss your bird before roasting, as the lemons fill the inside cavity while keeping the meat moist and providing a note of citrus.

One 3-pound chicken, giblets removed
2 lemons, quartered
1 sprig fresh rosemary

¼ cup pitted olives
4 anchovies packed in oil, rinsed under cold running water

10 ounces kale, trimmed, any variety (about 4 cups leaves)
1 tablespoon olive oil
Sea salt

Preheat the oven to 400°F. Rinse the chicken well under cold running water and pat dry with paper towels. Stuff the cavity with the lemons and rosemary and transfer the chicken to a roasting pan.

Place the olives and anchovies in a food processor and pulse until finely chopped. Carefully pull the skin of the chicken loose and press the olive mixture under the skin.

Transfer the chicken to the oven and roast for 45 minutes until the chicken skin starts to brown. Reduce the oven temperature to 350°F and continue to roast for 1 hour more, or until the chicken is no longer pink when pierced at the thigh joint and an instant-read thermometer registers 165°F. Transfer the chicken to a board and let rest for 5 minutes before carving.

While the chicken is cooking, prepare the kale. Place the kale in a large bowl along with the olive oil and toss well. Spread out onto two baking sheets, and lightly sprinkle with sea salt from 2 feet above the baking sheets. (Sea salt can be swapped out for red pepper flakes, curry powder, or other spices if desired.) During the last 10 minutes of roasting the chicken, transfer the baking sheets to the oven. Bake for 8 to 10 minutes until the edges of the kale are crisp. Serve immediately with the chicken.

NUTRITIONAL STATS PER SERVING (½ POUND MEAT AND 2 CUPS KALE): 391 Calories ❖ 51g protein (113%) ❖ 12g Carbohydrates ❖ 16g Fat (3g Saturated) ❖ 166mg Cholesterol ❖ 1g Sugars ❖ 4g Fiber ❖ 439mg Sodium

Vitamin C = 179% ❖ Protein = 113% ❖ Selenium = 80% ❖ Choline = 68% ❖ Zinc = 41%

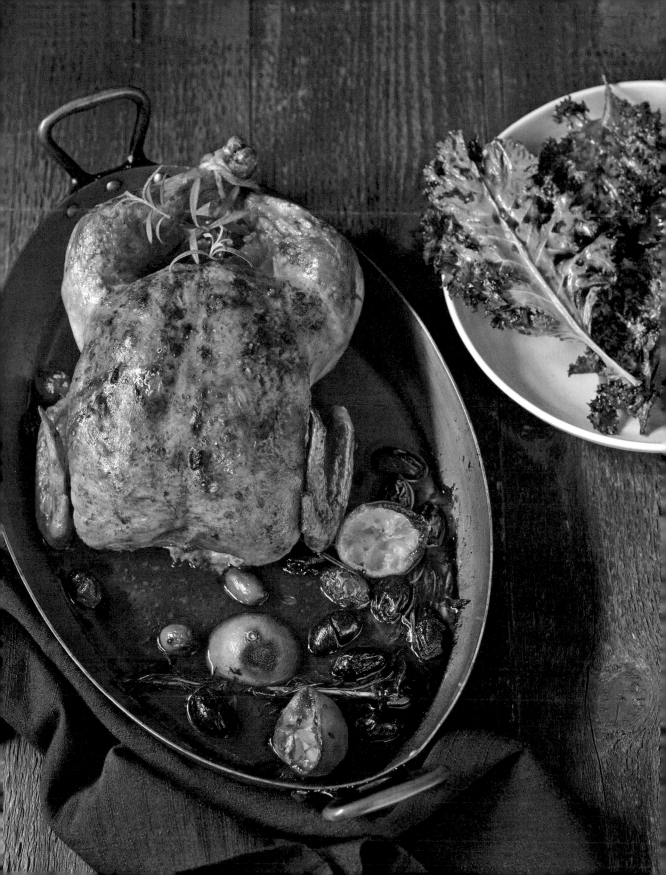

Roasted Pork Loin and Red Cabbage–Fennel Sauerkraut with Toasted Cumin Seed SERVES 4

Fear not the ferment! A key to eating complete is reaping the many benefits of fermented foods (see page 52). After a century of fighting against bacteria in every aspect of life, it's time to make peace with bugs and use them to keep your gut healthy and happy. It may seem a strange prescription to ferment cabbage in your kitchen, but sauerkraut is an approachable, simple ferment. The flavor pairs wonderfully with pork, which is the top source of thiamine (vitamin B), a nutrient required by your cells to make energy.

If you don't want to try your hand at fermenting your own sauerkraut, there are plenty of quality store-bought options. You can seek out real sauerkraut and other fermented vegetables at the local farmers' market or co-op, or try your local grocery store for lower-sodium options.

½ head red cabbage, thinly sliced or shredded

1 fennel bulb, trimmed

¼ cup raw apple cider vinegar

¼ teaspoon salt

One 2-pound pork loin

2 tablespoons handmade artisan jam, any flavor

1 tablespoon olive oil

2 teaspoons cumin seeds

Prepare the sauerkraut. Place the cabbage and fennel in a large bowl along with the vinegar and salt. With clean hands, squeeze the cabbage and fennel, working in the salt, for about 2 minutes until the mixture has released some of its liquid and decreases in size by about one-third. Transfer to a clean glass jar and press down with a spatula, then drizzle water over the surface. It's important that the cabbage remains submerged in its liquid during fermentation, to avoid mold and browning.

Cover the jar with a coffee filter or clean tea towel and secure with a rubber band to allow air in and keep debris out. Let rest on the countertop for 3 to 4 days, pressing the cabbage under the level of the water to allow it to ferment properly. The sauerkraut is safe to eat at every stage of the process, so fermentation time may vary depending on your tastes. Start tasting after day 5 for flavor. You may see bubbles, foam, or white scum on the surface of the sauerkraut, but these are all signs of normal, healthy fermentation. When your sauerkraut is fermented to your taste (or if you've opted for store-bought sauerkraut), cook the pork.

Preheat the oven to 400°F. Set the pork loin in a 7 × 11-inch baking dish. Put the jam and olive oil in a small bowl and mix with a fork. Brush over the pork and sprinkle with the cumin seeds. Transfer the pork to the oven and roast for 25 to 30 minutes until the meat is no longer pink/translucent inside and an instant-read thermometer inserted in the center registers at least 145°F. Serve alongside the sauerkraut.

NUTRITIONAL STATS PER SERVING (⅛ POUND PORK AND 1 CUP SAUERKRAUT): 199 Calories ❖ 27g Protein ❖ 10g Carbohydrates ❖ 5g Fat (2g Saturated) ❖ 168mg Cholesterol ❖ 4g Sugars ❖ 2g Fibe ❖ 95mg Sodium

Thiamine = 107% ❖ Selenium = 74% ❖ Protein = 59% ❖ Vitamin C = 45% ❖ Choline = 41%

Grilled Chicken with Asparagus-Almond-Tarragon Pesto SERVES 4

Make your grilled chicken a memorable, nutrient-rich experience. Lovers of traditional basil pesto will be pleased with this culinary twist, which calls for almonds (high in vitamin E) and asparagus (high in fiber and tryptophan). Tarragon is delectable with red meat, so make a double batch of this pesto and spoon some over grilled steak on another night. The pesto also makes a great dipping sauce for cookouts, parties, and any gatherings in need of more brain nutrients. Tarragon is a main herb in the Mediterranean diet and is one of the top plants in terms of antioxidant properties.

½ pound asparagus, trimmed
¼ cup olive oil
¼ cup fresh tarragon leaves
¼ cup almonds

2 garlic cloves
½ teaspoon salt
4 skinless, boneless chicken breasts

1 pound zucchini or yellow squash, trimmed and thinly sliced lengthwise

Preheat a grill over high heat.

Put the asparagus, olive oil, tarragon, almonds, garlic, and salt in a food processor and process until a chunky mixture forms. Divide the mixture in half, and spoon half of it onto the chicken breasts. Transfer the chicken to the grill and cook for 12 to 15 minutes, turning often, until the chicken is cooked through and no longer pink in the center.

While the chicken is cooking, brush the zucchini with the remaining pesto and place it on the grill. Grill for 4 to 5 minutes, turning often, until the zucchini is tender. Serve immediately with the chicken.

NUTRITIONAL STATS PER SERVING (1 BREAST AND 1 CUP VEGETABLES): 334 Calories ❖ 29g Protein ❖ 8g Carbohydrates ❖ 21g Fat (3g Saturated) ❖ 73mg Cholesterol ❖ 4g Sugars ❖ 3g Fiber ❖ 433mg Sodium

Selenium = 69% ❖ Protein = 63% ❖ Vitamin K = 41% ❖ Vitamin C, Choline = 33% ❖ Magnesium = 26%

Grass-Fed Beef Tenderloin with Pan-Roasted Apples and Fennel SERVES 4

Celebrate the bounty of fall with the flavor of apples at their prime. Using grass-fed beef means more nutrients (carotenoids, vitamin E, and conjugated linoleic acid), fewer calories, and true beef flavor. Being leaner meat, grass-fed cuts can overcook easily, so keep an eye on them. Not a fan of fennel? Substitute three thickly sliced red or Vidalia onions. Alternatively, serve the beef and apples with a side salad or grilled asparagus.

4 tablespoons coconut oil or unsalted grass-fed butter

2 apples, any variety, cored and sliced

2 fennel bulbs, trimmed and thinly sliced

1 teaspoon paprika or chipotle chile powder

½ teaspoon salt

Zest and juice of 1 lemon

4 grass-fed beef tenderloin center-cut filets mignons (6 ounces each)

½ teaspoon freshly ground black pepper

Preheat the oven to 400°F. Warm 2 tablespoons of the oil or batter in a large skillet over high heat. Add the apples, fennel, and paprika or chipotle chile powder, along with ¼ teaspoon of the salt. Reduce the heat to medium and cook for 10 to 12 minutes, stirring often, until the apples and fennel are tender. Stir in the lemon zest and juice. Set aside.

Sprinkle the filets with the black pepper and the remaining ¼ teaspoon salt. Heat a separate large skillet or cast-iron skillet over medium-high heat. Put in the remaining 2 tablespoons oil or butter and the filets. Cook for 3 to 4 minutes, without turning, until well seared, then turn and sear the opposite sides, 3 to 4 minutes. Slide the skillet with the filets into the oven and cook for 10 to 15 minutes until medium rare or medium according to your preference. Let rest 5 minutes, then serve with the apples and fennel.

NUTRITIONAL STATS PER SERVING (1 GRASS-FED FILET MIGNON AND 1 CUP APPLE-FENNEL MIX):
368 Calories ❖ 31g Protein ❖ 24g Carbohydrates ❖ 18g Fat (13g Saturated) ❖ 80mg Cholesterol ❖ 10g Sugars ❖ 7g Fiber ❖ 400mg sodium.

Vitamin B$_{12}$ = 158% ❖ Zinc = 89% ❖ Selenium = 73% ❖ Protein = 67% ❖ Vitamin C = 52%

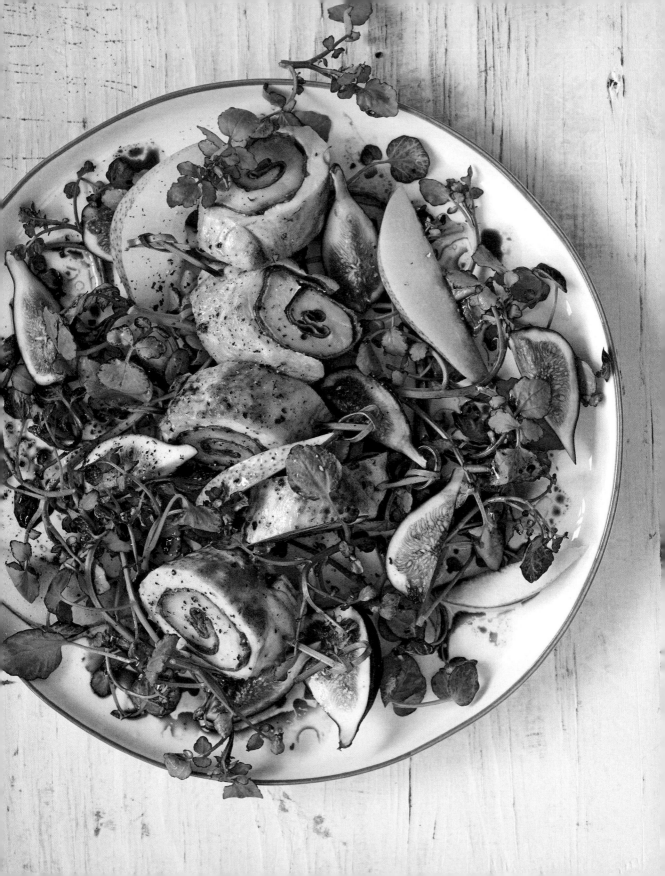

Collard and Prosciutto Chicken Roulades over Watercress Salad SERVES 4

This is a simple recipe that tends to impress. These elegant roulades are surprisingly easy to make and will get you a standing ovation at the dinner table. Take a bow, as you're giving everyone a nice dose of brain protection thanks to the vitamin A, vitamin C, vitamin K, fiber, and phytonutrients found in the watercress and collards. If you can't locate fresh figs, swap in two thinly sliced ripe pears, and feel free to swap out the collards for kale. Other salads in the book can be substituted for the watercress.

4 thinly sliced raw chicken cutlets (about 1 pound)

½ teaspoon paprika

½ teaspoon onion powder

¼ teaspoon freshly ground black pepper

4 slices prosciutto

4 large collard leaves, trimmed

4 tablespoons olive oil

1 pound watercress

2 tablespoons balsamic vinegar

1 pint fresh figs, quartered

Preheat the oven to 400°F. Set out all four chicken cutlets on a cutting board and sprinkle with the paprika, onion powder, and black pepper. Place a slice of the prosciutto on top of each chicken cutlet, then a collard leaf. Roll the stacks up, chicken on the outside, and secure with a toothpick.

Coat a large, oven-safe skillet with 1 tablespoon of the olive oil. Place over high heat and add the chicken roulades. Brown for 3 to 4 minutes, turning often. Transfer the skillet with the chicken to the oven and bake for 10 to 15 minutes until the chicken is cooked through. Transfer to a clean cutting board and let rest for 5 minutes.

Place the watercress in a large bowl along with the remaining 3 tablespoons oil and the vinegar and toss well to coat. Divide the watercress equally among four plates. Top with the figs. Slice the chicken and arrange over the watercress. Serve immediately.

NUTRITIONAL STATS PER SERVING (1 CHICKEN ROULADE, 2 CUPS SALAD): 305 Calories ❖ 35g Protein ❖ 11g Carbohydrates ❖ 13g Fat (2g Saturated) ❖ 87mg Cholesterol ❖ 7g Sugars ❖ 2g Fiber ❖ 427mg Sodium

Vitamin K = 474% ❖ Vitamin C = 80% ❖ Protein = 75% ❖ Selenium = 69% ❖ Vitamin A = 41%

Cast-Iron Steak Dinner with Buttery Cauliflower Mash SERVES 4

This recipe is a foolproof way to hear "Now that's a perfect steak!" Preheating the skillet is key, and cast iron is recommended—it gets hotter compared with other skillets, resulting in a nice sear. Ditch the traditional potatoes for this cauliflower mash for 75 percent fewer carbs and more vitamin C.

- 1 head cauliflower, cut into florets
- 4 garlic cloves, peeled and chopped
- 1/3 cup grass-fed whole milk
- 2 tablespoons unsalted grass-fed butter
- 1/2 teaspoon garlic salt
- 1/4 teaspoon freshly ground black pepper
- 1/4 teaspoon ground turmeric
- Four 8-ounce grass-fed steaks, such as shell steak, strip, rib eye, or flatiron
- 1/4 teaspoon salt
- 1/2 teaspoon freshly ground black pepper
- 1 tablespoon olive oil

Fit a large stockpot with a steamer basket, put in 2 inches of water, and bring to boil. Add the cauliflower florets, cover, and steam for 6 to 8 minutes until very tender when pierced with a fork. Set aside to cool for 4 to 5 minutes.

Put the garlic, milk, butter, garlic salt, pepper, and turmeric in a food processor along with the cooked cauliflower and process until smooth (you may need to do this in batches). Add a few tablespoons of warm water if the mixture doesn't blend smoothly, to adjust the consistency. Transfer the mixture back to the stockpot to keep warm while you prepare the steak.

Preheat the skillet over high heat for about 1 minute until very hot. Sprinkle the steak with the salt and black pepper. Put the oil in the skillet, then add the steak and cook for 6 to 8 minutes, turning once or twice, until a sear forms and the meat is medium rare. For a medium steak cook for 2 to 3 minutes more.

Transfer the steak to a cutting board and tent lightly with aluminum foil. Let rest 5 minutes. Serve with the cauliflower mash.

NUTRITIONAL STATS PER SERVING (ONE 8-OUNCE STEAK AND 1½ CUPS MASH): 401
Calories ❖ 56g Protein ❖ 9g Carbohydrates ❖ 16g Fat (6g Saturated) ❖ 142mg Cholesterol ❖ 3g Sugars ❖ 3g Fiber ❖ 443mg Sodium

Vitamin B$_{12}$ = 129% ❖ Vitamin C = 104% ❖ Protein = 100% ❖ Zinc = 99% ❖ Choline = 68%

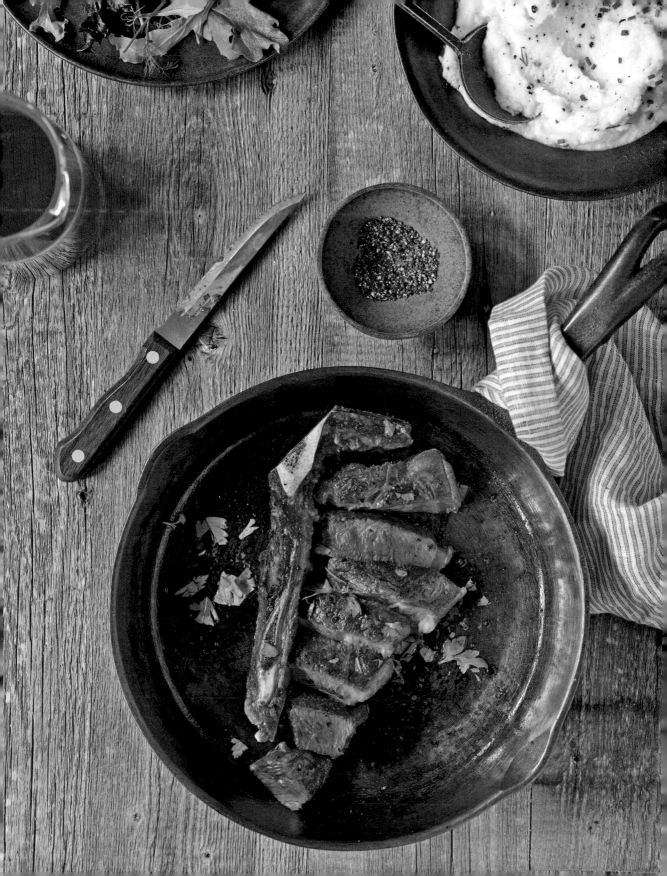

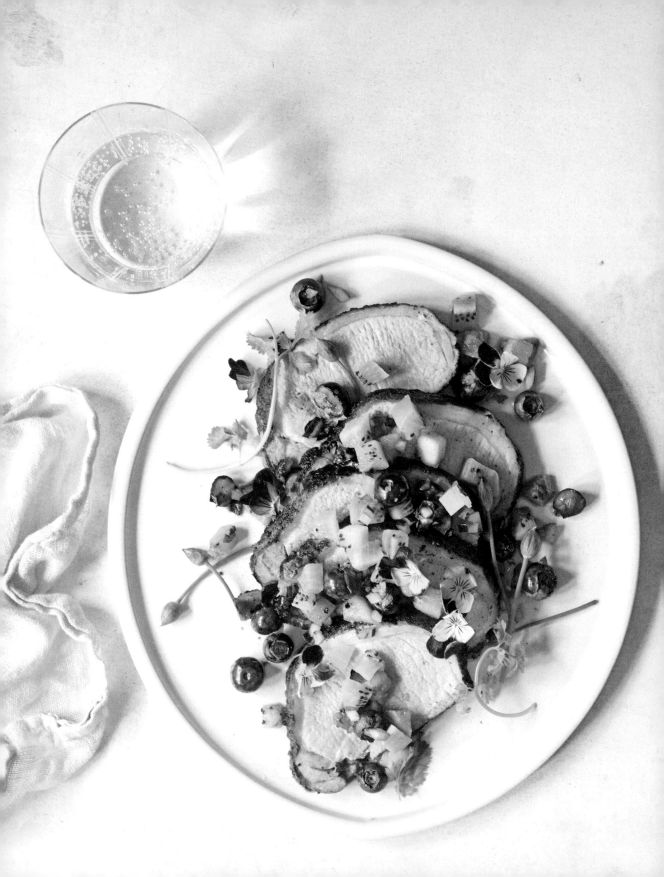

Chipotle Pork Loin with Blueberry-Kiwi Salsa SERVES 6

Tart kiwi and sweet blueberries make a unique salsa to dress your basic pork loin. This is a leaner cut of pork, so be sure not to overcook it; you can test the meat by slicing it with a paring knife or using an instant-read thermometer, which should register 145°F. Most pork tenderloins come in 2-pound portions, so if you're cooking for two, enjoy the leftovers or ask the butcher for a 1-pound portion.

2 kiwis, peeled and diced

1 pint blueberries, chopped

½ cup cilantro leaves, chopped

¼ cup minced red onion

2 tablespoons balsamic vinegar

1 teaspoon salt

¾ teaspoon paprika or chipotle chile powder

½ teaspoon ground turmeric

½ teaspoon ground cumin

¼ teaspoon freshly ground black pepper

One 2-pound center-cut pork loin

2 tablespoons grapeseed oil, plus more for the grill

To grill the pork loin, preheat a grill over high heat, or to roast, preheat the oven to 400°F.

Combine the kiwis, blueberries, cilantro, onion, and vinegar in a large bowl. Add ¼ teaspoon of the salt and toss well. Set the salsa aside.

Place the paprika or chipotle chile powder on a plate along with the turmeric, cumin, the remaining ¾ teaspoon salt, and the black pepper. Roll the pork loin in the spice mixture to coat. Drizzle the pork with the oil.

TO GRILL: Grease the grill with grapeseed oil. Adjust the grill flame setting to medium to medium-low. Place the loin on the grill and cook, turning often, until no longer translucent inside and cooked through, or until it registers 145°F on an instant-read thermometer, 20 to 25 minutes. Let the loin rest for 5 minutes before slicing, then serve with the salsa.

TO ROAST:. Place the pork in a 7 × 11-inch baking dish and roast on the lower rack, uncovered, for 35 to 40 minutes until cooked through and no longer pink in the center, and it registers 145°F on an instant-read thermometer. Let the loin rest for 5 minutes before slicing, then serve with the salsa.

NUTRITIONAL STATS PER SERVING (¼ POUND PORK WITH SALSA): 277 Calories ❖ 34g Protein ❖ 20g Carbohydrates ❖ 6g Fat (1g Saturated) ❖ 104mg Cholesterol ❖ 14g Sugars ❖ 3g Fiber ❖ 382mg Sodium

Selenium = 102% ❖ Thiamine = 76 ❖ Protein = 61% ❖ Vitamin C = 55% ❖ Zinc = 38%

Country Ribs with Honeyed Millet and Blood Oranges SERVES 4

Country ribs are a leaner, meatier option, which means you get more nutrients such as vitamin B$_{12}$, protein, and zinc for fewer calories. Look for them in a meat section where your standard pork cuts are sold. Since they are boneless, pay close attention to cooking time, to keep them tender and moist.

¼ cup organic ketchup

2 tablespoons apple cider vinegar

1 tablespoon brown sugar

½ teaspoon paprika

½ teaspoon chipotle chile powder

¼ teaspoon freshly ground black pepper

¼ teaspoon ground turmeric

¼ cup water

½ cup uncooked millet

¼ cup chopped fresh flat-leaf parsley

1 tablespoon honey

½ teaspoon Dijon mustard

Olive oil

12 boneless country pork ribs

1 tablespoon extra-virgin olive oil

2 quarts Brussels sprouts, trimmed and quartered

2 blood oranges, peeled and segmented

Preheat the oven to 400°F.

Combine the ketchup, vinegar, brown sugar, paprika, chipotle chile powder, black pepper, and turmeric along with the water in a small saucepan. Bring to a simmer over medium heat and cook for 10 to 15 minutes until thickened. Remove from the heat and set the barbecue sauce aside to cool.

Cook the millet according to the package instructions. Stir in the parsley, honey, and mustard and toss to combine. Set the millet aside.

Coat a 7 × 11-inch baking dish with the olive oil. Arrange the ribs in the dish and brush with the barbecue sauce. Transfer the ribs to the oven and bake for 25 to 35 minutes, brushing with additional sauce as needed. Test the ribs for doneness by slicing one with a paring knife. It should be cooked through and no longer pink in the center.

While the ribs are cooking, heat a large skillet over medium heat and put in the extra-virgin olive oil. Add the Brussels sprouts and cook for 4 to 5 minutes until they start to brown. Cook for 3 to 4 minutes more on low heat until they are crisp-tender.

Divide the millet equally among four plates and top with the Brussels sprouts. Top each plate with 3 ribs and a few segments of blood orange and serve immediately.

NUTRITIONAL STATS PER SERVING (3 RIBS WITH MILLET AND BRUSSELS SPROUTS): 412 Calories ❖ 33g Protein ❖ 52g Carbohydrates ❖ 10g Fat (2g Saturated) ❖ 55mg Cholesterol ❖ 20g Sugars ❖ 10g Fiber ❖ 438mg Sodium

Vitamin K = 350% ❖ Protein = 74% ❖ Fiber = 40% ❖ Folate = 38% ❖ Thiamine = 36%

Bacon Bison Burger with Pickles and Mustard SERVES 4

Bison is complemented in this dish by another lean, nutrient-dense meat: bacon. Bison, though similar to grass-fed beef, makes a flavorful burger that's also a cut above. If you can't find bison in your local grocery store you can order it frozen online to stock your freezer and save. Another option is to swap it out for another local meat, such as ground venison. Ensure healthier, higher-quality wraps by steering clear of those that have fake fats, colors, or preservatives listed in the ingredients. And when it comes to the bacon, try to buy local, pasture-raised, nitrate-free, smoked pork.

4 slices bacon
1 pound ground bison
¼ teaspoon salt
¼ teaspoon freshly ground black pepper
1 tablespoon olive oil
4 whole grain or gluten-free wraps
2 cups assorted greens
12 pickles
4 teaspoons Dijon mustard

Put the bacon in a small cold skillet and place over medium heat. Cook for 15 to 20 minutes, turning often, until crisp. Transfer to a paper towel to drain.

Combine the bison in a large bowl with the salt and the pepper. Form the bison into four 6-inch patties. Warm the oil in a large cast-iron skillet over medium-high heat. Add the burgers and cook for 8 to 10 minutes, turning once or twice, until the burgers are browned and cooked to medium inside.

Warm the wraps in the toaster oven for 2 to 3 minutes, or directly over a gas burner for 10 seconds.

Set out the wraps and top each with ½ cup of the greens, 3 of the pickles, and 1 teaspoon of the mustard. Top with a burger and a strip of bacon. Fold the wrap over and serve.

NUTRITIONAL STATS PER SERVING (1 BURGER WITH FIXINGS): 347 Calories ❖ 35g Protein ❖ 21g Carbohydrates ❖ 14g Fat (4g Saturated) ❖ 67mg Cholesterol ❖ 5g Sugars ❖ 1g Fiber ❖ 793mg Sodium

Vitamin K = 186% ❖ Vitamin B$_{12}$ = 98% ❖ Protein = 76% ❖ Zinc = 73% ❖ Selenium = 49%

Cinnamon-Fennel Brined Pork Chop with Cauliflower Hash SERVES 4

Overnight brining brings serious flavor to your standard pork chop. Potato hash fans will fall for this version made with cauliflower—a surprising source of vitamin C and potassium. This cruciferous vegetable is also very low in calories and doesn't come with the high starch load of a potato. Cooking time will vary depending on the thickness of your chops.

2 cinnamon sticks
1 teaspoon fennel seeds
1 teaspoon black peppercorns
¼ cup kosher salt

2 quarts water
4 grass-fed pork chops
½ teaspoon freshly ground black pepper
1 tablespoon grapeseed or coconut oil

2 tablespoons unsalted grass-fed butter
1 head cauliflower, cut into florets
½ red onion, peeled and minced

Place the cinnamon sticks, fennel seeds, and black pepper in a large saucepan along with the salt and 2 quarts water. Bring to a boil over high heat and stir well to dissolve the salt. Allow to cool to room temperature. Submerge the chops in the brine, making sure to leave space at the top. Cover with a lid and refrigerate for 10 to 12 hours.

When ready to cook, remove the chops from the brine and pat dry with paper towels. Sprinkle the pork shops with the ground pepper. Heat a large skillet over high heat and put in the oil. Add the chops and cook for 4 to 5 minutes per side, turning once or twice until the pork is no longer pink or translucent in the center.

While the pork is cooking, prepare the hash. Heat the butter in a separate large skillet over medium heat. Add the cauliflower and onion; cover; and cook for 10 to 12 minutes, stirring occasionally, until the cauliflower is well browned and the onion is soft. Serve immediately with the pork chops.

NUTRITIONAL STATS PER SERVING (1 PORK CHOP AND 1½ CUPS HASH): 347 Calories ❖ 35g Protein ❖ 21g Carbohydrates ❖ 14g Fat (4g Saturated) ❖ 67mg Cholesterol ❖ 5g Sugars ❖ 1g Fiber ❖ 793mg Sodium

Vitamin C = 97% ❖ Selenium = 62% ❖ Thiamine = 59% ❖ Protein = 76% ❖ Zinc = 42%

Pumpkin Seed–Crusted Lamb Chops with Red Lentil–Quinoa Pilaf SERVES 4

Grass-fed lamb is more flavorful compared with conventionally raised lamb, and it has become easier to find in recent years. This dish is ideal for a family celebration or a night when you want to treat yourself. If you aren't in the mood for pilaf, serve this lamb with the Pancetta Brussels Sprouts (see page 151).

½ cup chopped fresh flat-leaf parsley leaves
¼ cup pumpkin seeds
¼ cup grated Parmesan cheese
½ teaspoon paprika
¼ teaspoon freshly ground black pepper

1 egg white, preferably from a pasture-raised egg
8 grass-fed lamb chops, about 1 pound
⅓ cup uncooked red lentils
½ cup uncooked quinoa or millet

3 cups vegetable broth, low-sodium chicken broth, or bone broth (see page 200)
1 tablespoon unsalted grass-fed butter, or olive oil
1 teaspoon fresh thyme leaves

Preheat the oven to 400°F.

Put the parsley, pumpkin seeds, Parmesan, paprika, and pepper in a food processor and pulse until a chunky mixture forms. Transfer to a plate.

Whisk the egg white in a shallow bowl.

Dip the chops in the beaten egg white and then press into the parsley mixture. Transfer the chops to baking sheets, a cast-iron skillet, or an ovenproof dish and into the oven. Bake for 20 to 25 minutes until the lamb is cooked through. Let it rest on the counter for 10 minutes. The meat will be pink in the center yet tender and easy to cut.

While the lamb is cooking, prepare the pilaf. Put the lentils, quinoa or millet, broth, butter or oil, and thyme in a small saucepan. Place over high heat and bring to a boil. Cover and reduce the heat to a simmer. Cook for 15 to 20 minutes until the lentils and grains are tender. Serve the lamb chops with the pilaf.

NUTRITIONAL STATS PER SERVING (2 CHOPS AND 1¼ CUPS PILAF): 488 Calories ❖ 37g Protein ❖ 25g Carbohydrates ❖ 26g Fat (11g Saturated) ❖ 87mg Cholesterol ❖ 1g Sugars ❖ 7g Fiber ❖ 457mg Sodium

Vitamin K = 141% ❖ Vitamin B$_{12}$ = 133% ❖ Protein = 80% ❖ Zinc = 75% ❖ Iron = 69%

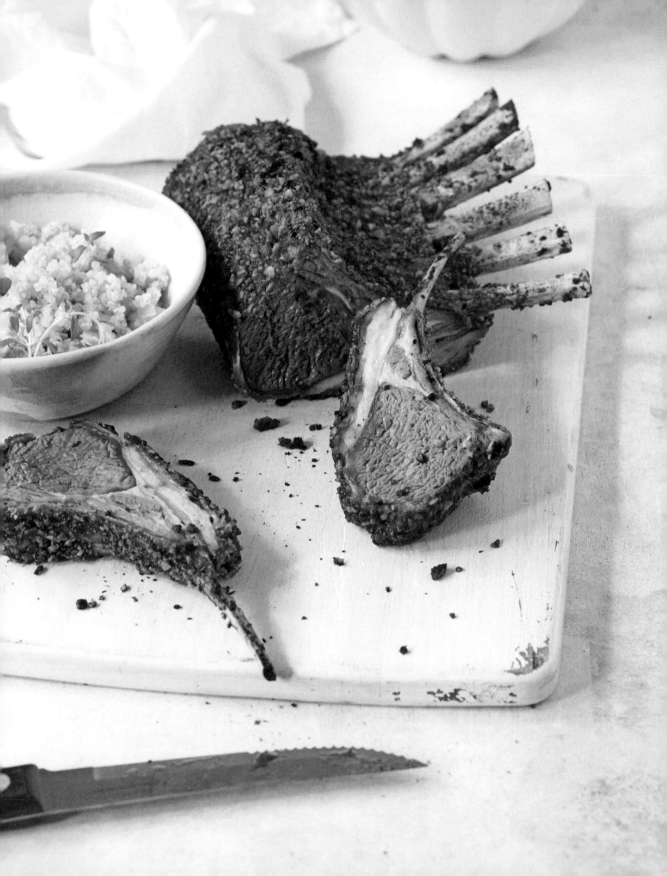

Lentil and Mushroom Shepherd's Pie with Sweet Potato Topping SERVES 6

This is serious nutrition packed into a one-dish comfort meal. For a shortcut, use canned organic sweet potato. More lentils mean more folate—a cup of these legumes has 90 percent of your daily need. And more folate means more happiness, mental clarity, and relaxation.

½ cup uncooked lentils

3 pounds sweet potatoes (about 3 large potatoes), peeled and quartered

1 tablespoon olive oil

1 medium onion, chopped (about 1½ cups)

One 5-ounce container mushrooms, such as cremini, button, or shiitake, chopped

1 pound grass-fed ground beef

1 tablespoon Worcestershire sauce

¼ teaspoon freshly ground black pepper, or other seasoning of choice

⅔ cup buttermilk or whole milk, preferably from grass-fed cows

1 teaspoon garlic powder

1 teaspoon baking powder

Cook the lentils according to the package instructions and set aside. Preheat the oven to 400°F.

Put the potatoes in a medium pot, cover with at least 1 inch of cold water, and bring to a boil. Reduce to a simmer and cook until tender, 12 to 15 minutes.

While the potatoes are cooking, warm the oil in a large skillet over medium heat. Add the chopped onion and mushrooms and cook until tender, 5 to 6 minutes.

Push the vegetables to the side and add the beef. Cook the beef for 2 to 3 minutes without moving it, to allow the beef to brown. Continue to cook, breaking up the meat, for about 2 minute more. Stir in the Worcestershire sauce, pepper, and lentils. Transfer to a 7 × 11-inch baking dish.

Once the potatoes are fork-tender, drain and transfer to a food processor along with the buttermilk and the garlic powder. Process until smooth. Sprinkle the baking powder over the mixture and process again to incorporate. Using a spatula, spoon the potato mixture over the meat mixture in the baking dish. Bake for 35 to 40 minutes until the pie is bubbling hot and the topping is golden. Let cool 5 minutes before serving.

NUTRITIONAL STATS PER SERVING (1¼ CUPS):
372 Calories ❖ 23g Protein ❖ 43g Carbohydrates ❖ 11g Fat (5g Saturated) ❖ 59mg Cholesterol ❖ 7g Sugars ❖ 10g Fiber ❖ 396mg Sodium

Vitamin A = 158% ❖ Vitamin B$_{12}$ = 71% ❖ Zinc = 61% ❖ Protein = 50% ❖ Fiber = 40%

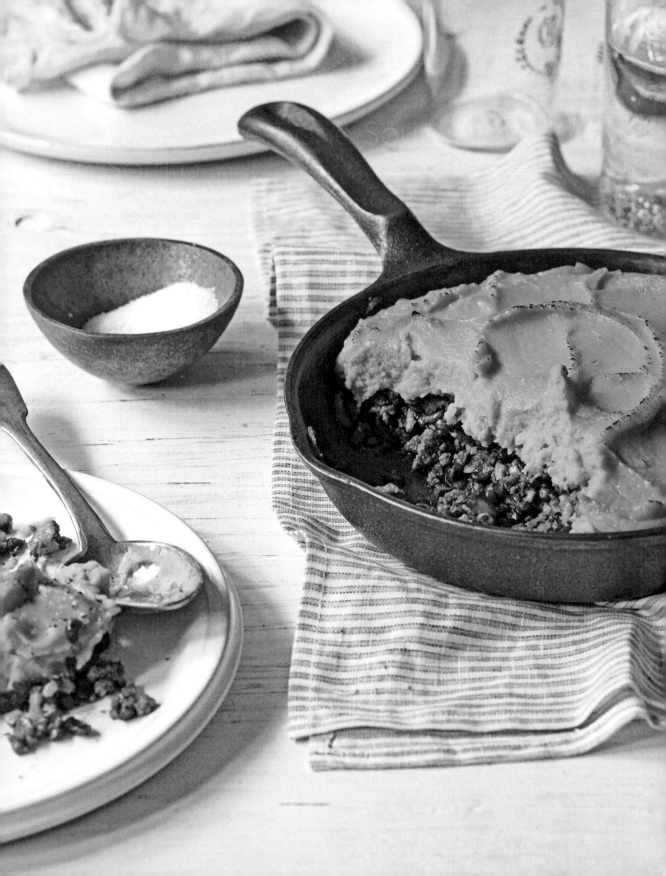

Sunday Slow-Cooker Beef Shank SERVES 8

Beef shanks make a great cut for this quickly prepped, slow-cooked meal. Stew lovers will enjoy it because it's a sophisticated version of braised beef that uses wine. During cooking, the alcohol in the wine will burn off, but you can use more water instead of wine if you prefer. You can also prepare this in a slow cooker—just sear the beef as instructed below, then place all the veggies and liquid along with the shank in a slow cooker on low for 6 to 8 hours.

¼ cup gluten-free oat flour
½ teaspoon paprika
½ teaspoon garlic powder
¼ teaspoon freshly ground black pepper
4 cross-cut, bone-in beef shanks (about 2½ pounds total)
2 tablespoons extra-virgin olive oil
1 medium onion, peeled and diced

4 carrots, peeled and diced
2 parsnips, peeled and diced
2 celery stalks, diced
4 medium garlic cloves, finely chopped
2 tablespoons tomato paste
½ cup dry white or red wine
2 cups bone broth (see page 200) or water
1 tablespoon balsamic vinegar

½ teaspoon dried oregano
4 sprigs fresh thyme

Gremolata
½ cup finely chopped fresh flat-leaf parsley
1 tablespoon finely grated zest from 1 or 2 lemons
2 medium garlic cloves, minced (about 2 teaspoons)

Place the oat flour, paprika, garlic powder, and pepper on a plate and mix with your fingertips. Press the beef shanks into the flour mixture.

Warm the oil in a large stockpot or braising pot over medium heat. Brown the beef shanks in batches, 8 to 10 minutes per batch, until an even crust forms on the shanks. Transfer all the shanks to a plate while you cook the veggies.

Add the onion, carrots, parsnips, celery, and the 4 garlic cloves to the pot and cook

for 4 to 5 minutes, stirring well, until the vegetables are tender. Add the tomato paste and cook for 1 minute more until fragrant. Carefully add the wine and cook for 2 to 3 minutes until reduced by half.

Return the shanks to the pot; add the stock, balsamic vinegar, oregano, and thyme; and bring to a boil. Cover, reduce the heat to low, and simmer for 2 to 2½ hours until the shanks are tender. Check the level of the liquid periodically during the simmer to make sure the liquid just covers the meat for the first 1½ hours of cooking. Add water in ¼-cup amounts if the liquid level drops too low.

While the shanks are cooking, make the gremolata. Put the parsley, lemon zest, and the 2 garlic cloves in a medium bowl and stir well.

Plate the shanks and vegetables, top with the gremolata, and serve immediately.

NUTRITIONAL STATS PER SERVING (½ SHANK AND VEGETABLES): 285 Calories ❖ 26g Protein ❖ 17g Carbohydrate ❖ 8g Fat (4g Saturated) ❖ 90mg Cholesterol ❖ 6g Sugars ❖ 4g Fiber ❖ 271mg Sodium

Vitamin B$_{12}$ = 315% ❖ Zinc = 200% ❖ Vitamin K = 153% ❖ Protein = 124% ❖ Selenium = 78%

Pan-Roasted Duck and Potatoes with Cherry Sauce SERVES 4

Savory duck with cherries will be a hit at your next dinner party or romantic evening in. This meatier poultry has four times the iron of chicken and delivers an intriguing mix of fats. Wild duck is a great way to mix things up for beef lovers. Find a local, organic bird if you can—from your local gourmet market or farmers' market. This dish pairs well with a chilled Rioja or Côtes du Rhône.

Olive oil

2 garlic cloves, thinly sliced

1 cup pitted sweet cherries, frozen or fresh

½ cup water

½ teaspoon pure vanilla extract

4 duck breasts, fat cap trimmed ¼ inch

½ teaspoon salt

¼ teaspoon freshly ground black pepper

½ pound tricolor, Red Bliss, or small creamer potatoes, halved

1 pound thin asparagus spears, ends trimmed

¼ cup microgreens (optional)

Preheat the oven to 400°F.

Coat a small saucepan with olive oil and add the garlic. Place over medium heat and cook for 2 to 3 minutes until the garlic starts to brown. Carefully add the cherries along with the water, cover, and cook for 4 to 5 minutes until the cherries soften. Add the vanilla and set aside to cool for 5 minutes. Using an immersion blender or stand blender, process until a smooth thick sauce forms. Set aside.

Score the fat side of the duck breasts with a sharp knife, making a crisscross mark over the surface; do not pierce the meat. Sprinkle the duck breasts with half the salt and pepper. Place the duck breasts in a cold, oven-safe skillet, fat side down; do not heat the skillet first—you want to render the fat slowly. Place the skillet over medium-high heat and cook the duck breasts for 2 to 3 minutes until the fat starts to melt and render out.

Reduce the heat to medium and continue to cook the duck breasts for 7 to 8 minutes until crisp. Turn and cook for another 4 to 5 minutes until browned. Pour off any excess fat and reserve for cooking the potatoes. Transfer the skillet to the oven and cook for 5 to 6 minutes for medium rare and 7 to 8 minutes for medium. Let the duck breasts rest on a carving board for 5 minutes to allow the juices to redistribute.

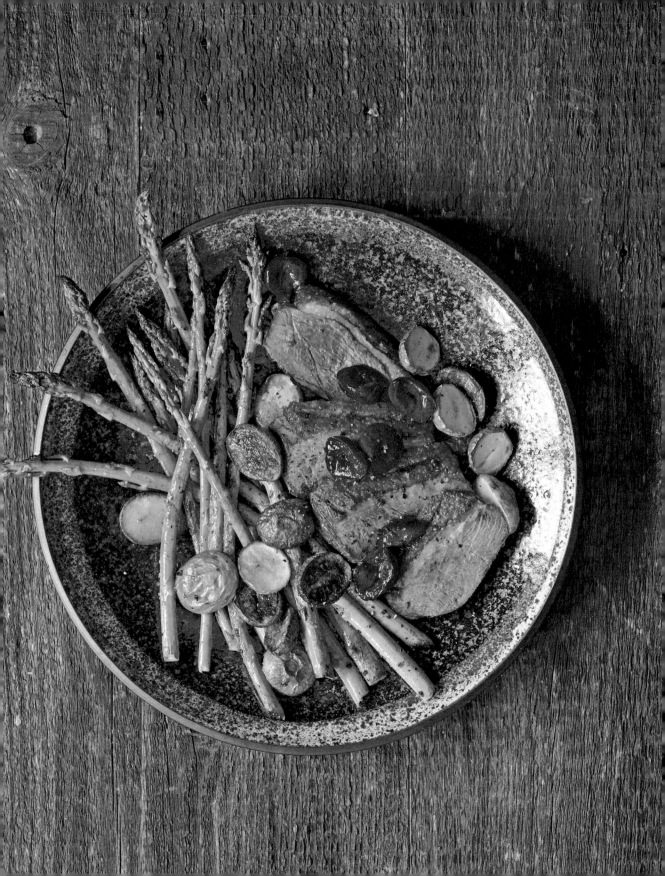

While the duck is cooking prepare the potatoes. Heat the reserved duck fat in a separate skillet over medium heat. Add the potatoes and season with the remaining salt and pepper. Cook for 10 to 12 minutes, turning occasionally, until the potatoes are golden brown. Reduce the heat to low; cover; and cook for 3 to 4 minutes more, or until the potatoes are tender. Set aside.

Coat a large skillet with olive oil and place over high heat. Add the asparagus and cook for 6 to 7 minutes until the spears start to soften and brown. Reduce the heat to low, cover, and cook for 3 to 4 minutes more until the spears are tender.

Slice the duck breasts and distribute among four plates. Drizzle with the sauce and garnish with the microgreens, if using. Serve with the potatoes and asparagus.

NUTRITIONAL STATS PER SERVING (1 DUCK BREAST, 5 MINI POTATOES, ¼ POUND ASPARAGUS): 409 Calories ❖ 37g protein ❖ 20g Carbohydrates ❖ 20g Fat (6g Saturated) ❖ 140mg Cholesterol ❖ 8g Sugars ❖ 4g Fiber ❖ 399mg Sodium

Thiamine = 82% ❖ Protein = 80% ❖ Vitamin K = 61% ❖ Iron = 58% ❖ Vitamin B$_{12}$ = 54%

Seafood

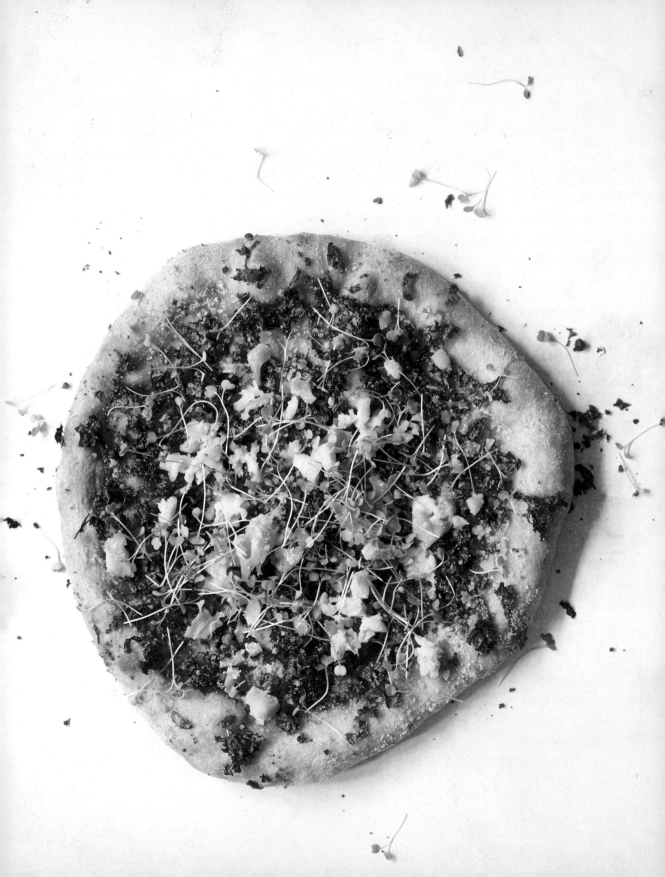

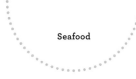

Rocket Pie SERVES 4

Feed your brain and tone your body with pizza? The fresh arugula, a.k.a. "rocket," that tops this pie adds a spicy bite to a rich, savory base. Clams contain more vitamin B_{12} than any other food and deliver protein, iron, and iodine. Higher levels of B_{12} in your blood mean a bigger, healthier brain as you age. You can pull this recipe off in just minutes by using dough from the freezer section in your grocery store and swapping out the fresh clams for jarred. Remember to place the dough in your fridge the night before to gently defrost.

½ pound clams, well rinsed under cold running water

6 tablespoons olive oil

2 garlic cloves

¼ teaspoon salt

2 cups packed kale leaves

½ pound frozen pizza dough (whole wheat or gluten-free), defrosted

½ cup grated pecorino Romano cheese

1 cup baby arugula or microgreens

Preheat the oven to 450°F.

Partially fill a large stockpot with 3 inches water and bring to a boil over high heat, Add the clams, cover, and cook for 2 to 3 minutes or until the shells open and the clams are cooked through inside. Drain and pull the clam meat from the shells. Chop the clams and set aside.

Place the olive oil, garlic, and salt in a food processor and pulse until finely chopped. Add the kale and pulse again until a chunky mixture forms.

Roll out the dough and place it on a pizza pan or baking sheet. Top with the kale mixture and, using the back of a spoon, spread it almost to the edges of the dough. Sprinkle with the clams and cheese. Bake for 15 to 20 minutes until the edges are cooked and golden. Remove from the oven and sprinkle with the arugula. Serve immediately.

NUTRITIONAL STATS PER SERVING (2 THIN SLICES): 408 Calories ❖ 17g Protein ❖ 30g Carbohydrates ❖ 26g Fat (5g Saturated) ❖ 26mg Cholesterol ❖ 0g Sugars ❖ 1g Fiber ❖ 759mg Sodium

Vitamin B_{12} = 276% ❖ Vitamin C = 60% ❖ Protein = 37% ❖ Selenium = 36% ❖ Iodine = 25%

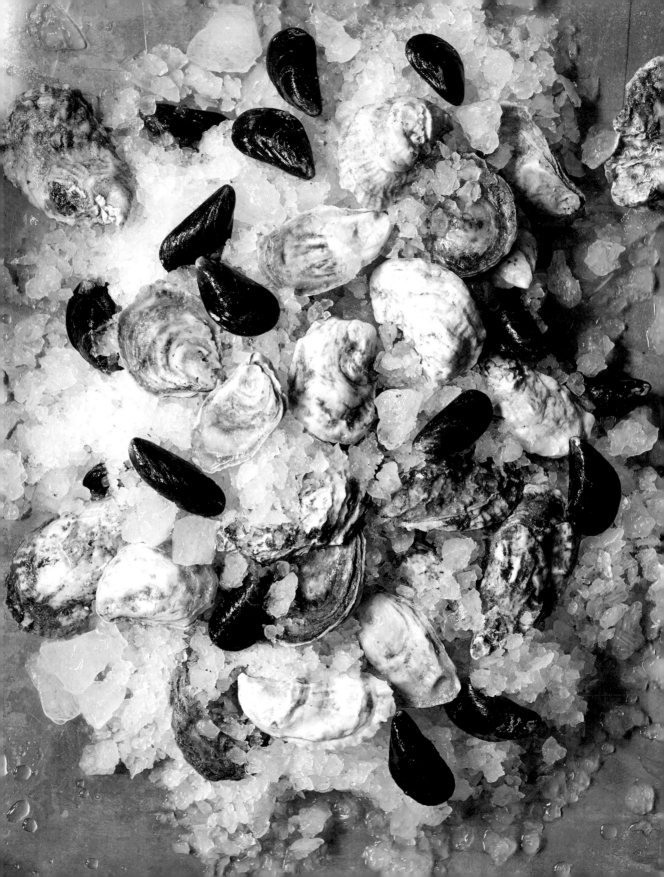

Mussels Three Ways ALL VERSIONS SERVE 4

1. With Heirloom Tomatoes and Pine Nut Topping
2. With Garlicky Kale Ribbons and Artichokes
3. With White Wine and Roasted Red Pepper

Mussels offer excellent nutrient density at a great value, making them an extremely accessible seafood. Avoid gritty mussels by soaking and rinsing them first, which allows tightly closed mussels to release any residual grit that the careless cook can miss. Because they're still alive, mussels are some of the freshest seafood in most stores.

Heirloom Tomatoes and Pine Nut Topping

1 tablespoon olive oil

½ onion, minced

4 tomatoes, diced

2 pounds wild or farm-raised raw, tightly closed mussels

1 cup low-sodium chicken, vegetable, or beef broth

½ cup chopped fresh basil

½ cup pine nuts

Garlicky Kale Ribbons and Artichokes

1 tablespoon olive oil

½ onion, minced

4 garlic cloves, thinly sliced

2 pounds wild or farm-raised raw, tightly closed mussels

4 large kale leaves, thinly sliced into ribbons

4 artichoke hearts, chopped

1 cup low-sodium chicken, vegetable, or beef broth

White Wine and Roasted Red Pepper

1 tablespoon olive oil

1 onion, minced

2 pounds wild or farm-raised raw, tightly closed mussels

½ cup white wine

¾ cup low-sodium chicken, vegetable, or beef broth

2 cups diced roasted red pepper

PREPARING MUSSELS FOR COOKING: Soak the mussels in a large bowl of cold water for 15 to 20 minutes. Using your fingers or a slotted spoon, lift out the mussels and transfer them to a colander. Rinse under cold running water several times and discard any mussels that are damaged or remain open after being firmly squeezed between your thumb and forefinger, or when you firmly tap them.

Check each mussel for a threadlike string hanging out of the shell (called the "beard"). To remove, use a tea towel to grasp the beard, and pull firmly towards the hinge end of the shell and tug free.

HEIRLOOM TOMATOES AND PINE NUT TOPPING: Warm the olive oil in a large stockpot over medium heat. Add the onion and cook for 3 to 4 minutes until the onion begins to brown. Add the tomatoes and

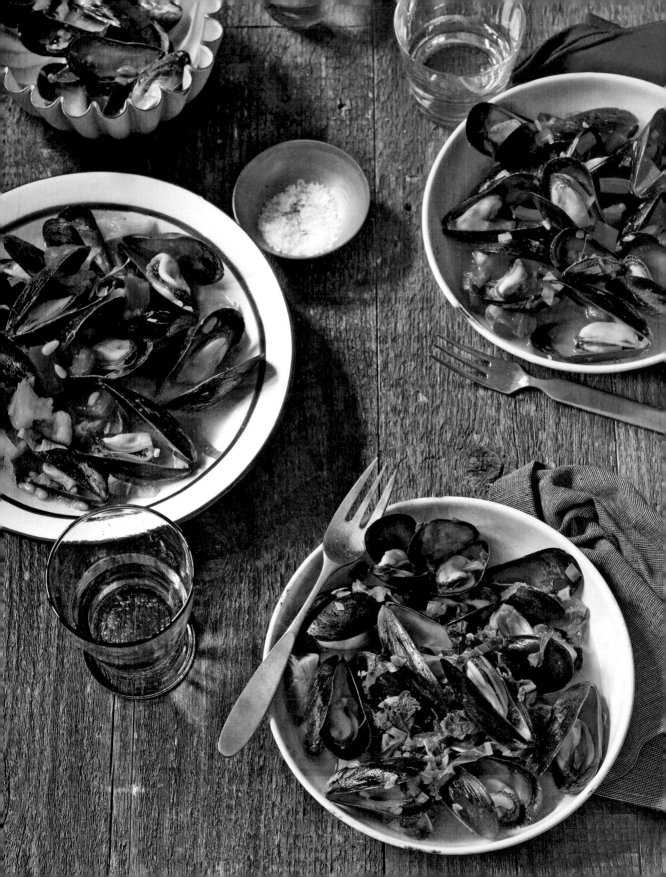

cook for 1 minute more until they begin to give off their liquid. Add the mussels and the broth. Cover and cook for 3 to 4 minutes until the mussels open and the meat inside is cooked through. Discard any mussels that have not opened. Sprinkle with the basil and pine nuts and serve immediately.

GARLICKY KALE RIBBONS AND ARTICHOKES: Warm the olive oil in a large stockpot over medium heat. Add the onion and garlic and cook for 3 to 4 minutes until the onion begins to brown. Add the mussels, kale, artichokes, and broth. Cover and cook 3 to 4 minutes until the mussels open and the meat inside is cooked through. Discard any mussels that have not opened. Serve immediately.

WHITE WINE AND ROASTED RED PEPPER: Warm the olive oil in a large stockpot over medium heat. Add the onion and cook for 3 to 4 minutes until the onion begins to brown. Add the mussels, wine, and broth. Cover and cook for 3 to 4 minutes until the muscles open and the meat inside is cooked through. Discard any mussels that have not opened. Sprinkle with the roasted red pepper and serve immediately.

HEIRLOOM TOMATOES AND PINE NUT TOPPING NUTRITIONAL STATS PER SERVING (½ POUND MUSSELS): 358 Calories ✤ 30g Protein ✤ 14g Carbohydrates ✤ 20g Fat (2g Saturated) ✤ 63mg Cholesterol ✤ 3g Sugars ✤ 2g Fiber ✤ 653mg Sodium

Vitamin B$_{12}$ = 1,133% ✤ DHA+EPA = 200% ✤ Selenium = 185% ✤ Protein = 67% ✤ Zinc = 61%

GARLICKY KALE RIBBONS AND ARTICHOKES NUTRITIONAL STATS PER SERVING (½ POUND MUSSELS): 334 Calories ✤ 33g Protein ✤ 32g Carbohydrates ✤ 9g Fat (2g Saturated) ✤ 63mg Cholesterol ✤ 4g Sugars ✤ 12g Fiber ✤ 750mg Sodium

Vitamin B$_{12}$ = 1,125% ✤ Vitamin K = 631% ✤ DHA+EPA = 200% ✤ Selenium = 187% ✤ Vitamin C = 147%

WHITE WINE AND ROASTED RED PEPPER NUTRITIONAL STATS PER SERVING (½ POUND MUSSELS): 266 Calories ✤ 28g Protein ✤ 13g Carbohydrates ✤ 9g Fat (1g Saturated) ✤ 63mg Cholesterol ✤ 2g Sugars ✤ 1g Fiber ✤ 652mg Sodium

Vitamin B$_{12}$ = 1,125% ✤ DHA+EPA = 200% ✤ Selenium = 185% ✤ Vitamin C = 77% ✤ Protein = 61%

Raw Oysters with Lemony Kale Drizzle SERVES 6

The original brain food is just 10 calories a pop. Oysters bring the top nutrients that so many people miss: vitamin B$_{12}$, zinc, iron, the long-chained omega-3 fats, and vitamin D. Opt for this lemony kale drizzle in place of cocktail sauce for a new alternative; plus, the combination of the salty brine with a tangy topping is a flavor delight. For spice lovers, double the crushed red pepper flakes or stir ¼ teaspoon ground cayenne directly into the drizzle before dressing your oysters.

2 cups packed kale leaves, chopped
½ cup fresh flat-leaf parsley or basil leaves

Finely grated zest of 1 lemon
1 tablespoon red wine vinegar
2 garlic cloves, halved

¼ teaspoon crushed red pepper flakes (optional)
¼ cup extra-virgin olive oil
18 raw oysters, shucked

Place the kale, parsley or basil, lemon zest, vinegar, garlic, and red pepper flakes, if using, in a food processor. Process until finely chopped. With the motor running add the olive oil and process until a smooth dressing forms. Drizzle over the oysters and serve immediately.

NUTRITIONAL STATS PER SERVING
(3 OYSTERS WITH DRESSING): 121 calories ❖
4g Protein ❖ 4g Carbohydrates ❖ 10g Fat (2g
Saturated) ❖ 22mg Cholesterol ❖ 1g Sugars ❖
1g Fiber ❖ 67mg sodium.

Vitamin B$_{12}$ = 204% ❖ Zinc = 280% ❖
Vitamin K = 98% ❖ Vitamin C = 48% ❖
DHA+EPA = 35%

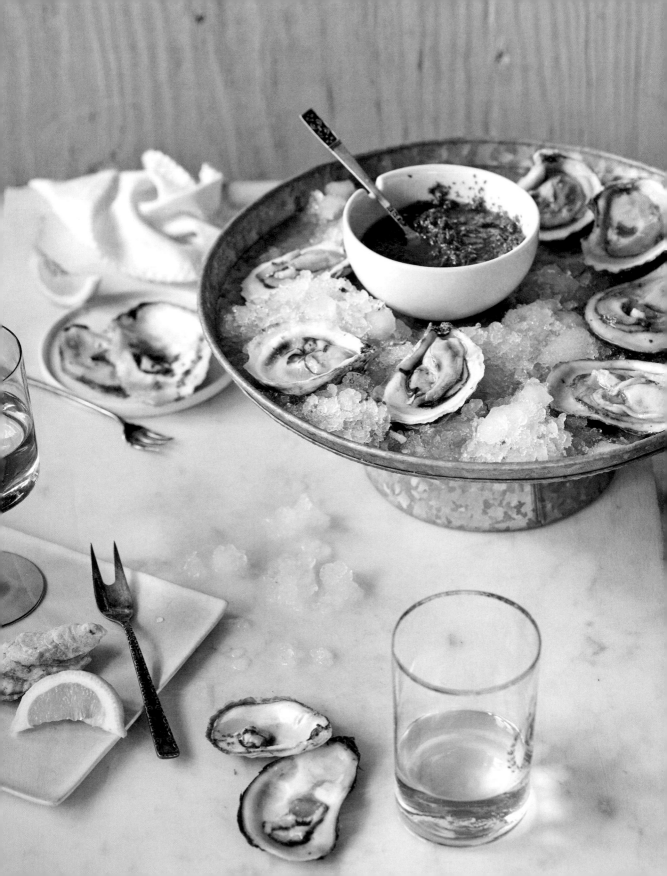

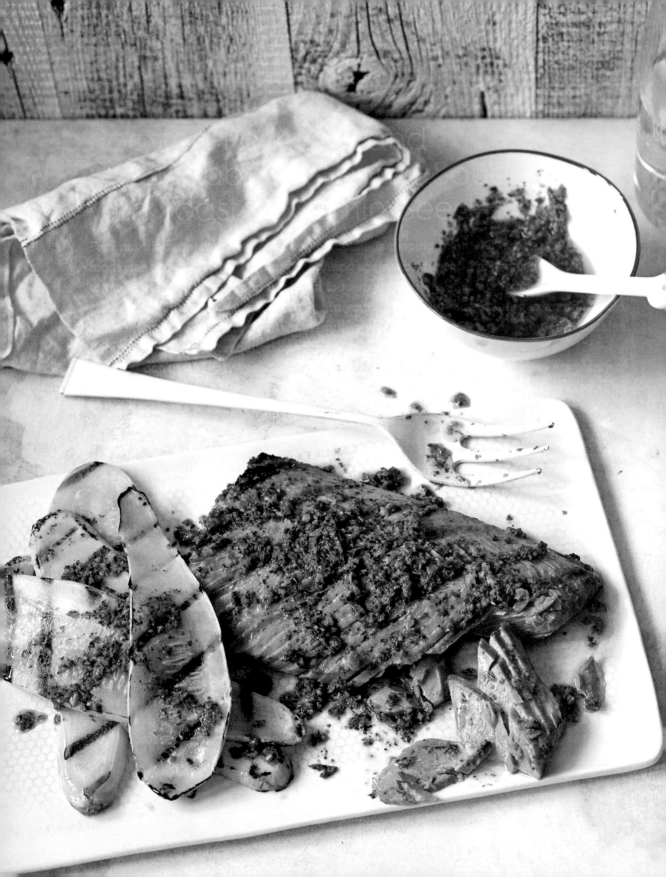

Grilled Wild Salmon with Garlic Scape Pesto and Summer Squash SERVES 4

Wild salmon tops the list of fish that are high in omega-3 and low in mercury. So swap out farmed salmon, which contains food dyes, for the real thing. Frozen sides of wild salmon offer the best value. Garlic scapes are the young, soft stems and unopened flower buds of hardneck garlic. This variety of garlic tends to be prevalent at farmers' markets. The season for scapes is short—just a few weeks in June—so if you can't find them you can substitute scallions or baby leeks.

Coconut oil, for the grill
2 cups garlic scapes
2 cups packed kale leaves
½ cup olive oil

½ cup grated Parmesan or pecorino Romano cheese
¼ teaspoon salt
⅛ teaspoon freshly ground black pepper

4 wild salmon fillets, skin intact (1 pound)
1 pound yellow squash, sliced into ¼-inch strips

Oil a grill with coconut oil and preheat the grill over high heat.

Put the garlic scapes, kale, olive oil, cheese, salt, and pepper in a food processor or blender and process until finely chopped. Divide the pesto in half and reserve one-half for another use.

Place the salmon on the grill, flesh side down, and grill 3 to 4 minutes. Turn the salmon, and place the squash slices on the grill. Brush the pesto over the salmon and the squash.

Grill the squash, turning it occasionally, for 4 to 5 minutes until cooked through. Grill the salmon 4 to 5 minutes until the skin crisps but the center is still medium. Transfer to a plate and serve immediately.

NUTRITIONAL STATS PER SERVING (1 SALMON FILLET AND 1 CUP SQUASH): 408 Calories ❖ 30g Protein ❖ 21g Carbohydrates ❖ 22g Fat (4g Saturated) ❖ 55mg Cholesterol ❖ 8g Sugars ❖ 2g Fiber ❖ 388mg Sodium

DHA+EPA = 246% ❖ Vitamin B$_{12}$, Vitamin D = 200% ❖ Selenium = 78% ❖ Vitamin C = 72% ❖ Protein = 67%

Garlic Butter Shrimp over Spiralized Zucchini SERVES 4

Shredding raw zucchini using a mandolin or spiralizer creates a nutrient-dense, low-sugar, gluten-free swap for pasta. Don't cut the zucchini noodles in advance, since they can become soggy and lose their firm texture. If you have yellow summer squash, it works equally well in this quick seafood dish. Avoid excess sodium by purchasing wild shrimp, which is not treated with the salt preservative common in farmed and frozen shrimp that elevates the sodium 4 to 5 times.

2 large zucchini (about 1½ pounds)

4 carrots, peeled

1 tablespoon coconut oil

1 pound medium wild shrimp, peeled and deveined

4 garlic cloves, minced

4 tablespoons unsalted grass-fed butter

¼ cup chopped fresh flat-leaf parsley

Shred the zucchini and carrots, using a Japanese mandolin or spiralizer, to make noodles. Set aside.

Heat a large skillet over high heat. Put in the coconut oil and the shrimp and cook for 2 to 3 minutes, stirring often, until the shrimp turn pink. Add the garlic and cook for 1 minute more until fragrant.

Add the zucchini and carrot noodles, reduce the heat to low, and toss well to distribute. Add the butter and cook for 1 minute until melted.

Serve immediately, garnished with the chopped parsley.

NUTRITIONAL STATS PER SERVING (¼ POUND SHRIMP WITH 2 CUPS NOODLES): 309 Calories ❖ 26g Protein ❖ 13g Carbohydrates ❖ 17g Fat (9g Saturated) ❖ 170mg Cholesterol ❖ 7g Sugars ❖ 4g Fiber ❖ 230mg Sodium

EPA+DHA 124% ❖ Selenium 100% ❖ Vitamin A 75% ❖ Protein 57% ❖ Vitamin C 53%

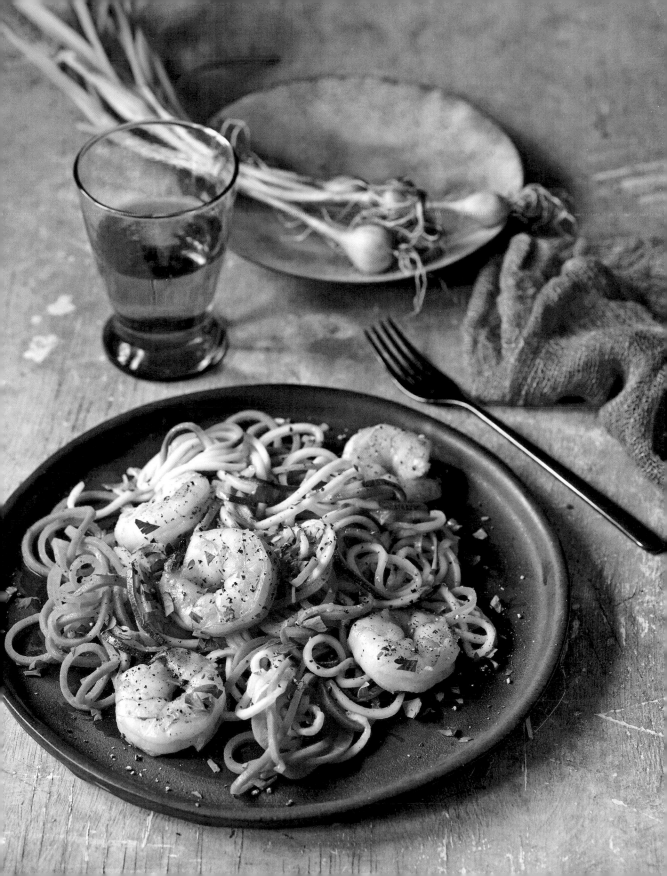

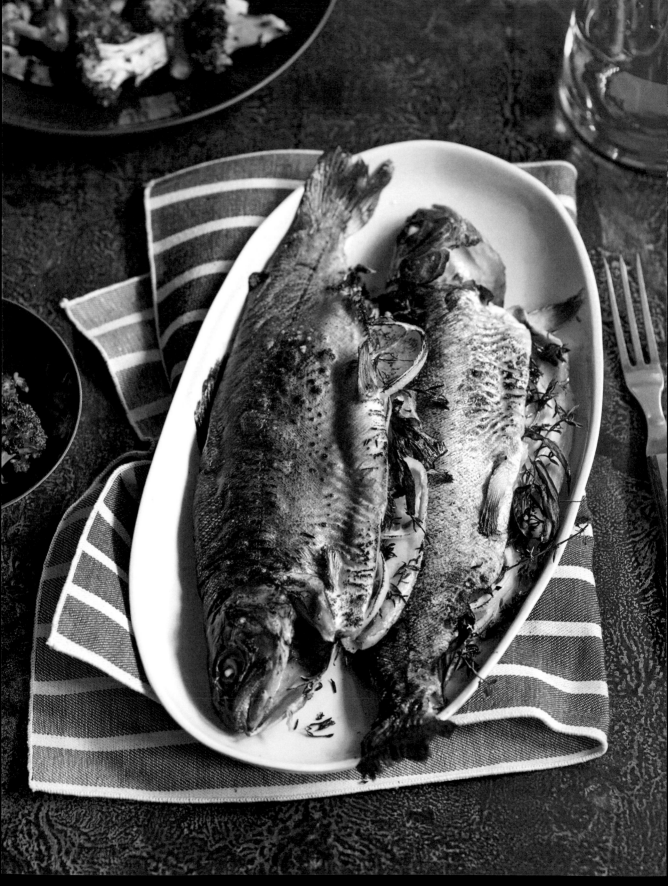

Whole Trout en Papillote with Garlic Broccoli SERVES 4

Steaming fish in parchment paper with quick-cooking vegetables and herbs is a simple and elegant way to cook and enjoy whole fish. It stays fresher longer compared with fillets in raw form, and the meat falls away easily from the bone after it is cooked. Trout is affordable and contains more omega-3 fats than most mild, white fish. Anchovies are also an affordable source of omega-3s for this dish. Watch your fingers for hot steam as you open the package; wearing kitchen gloves is a useful trick for ease of handling before you dig in.

4 whole trout, cleaned (about 1½ pounds)

4 tablespoons olive oil

½ teaspoon salt

½ teaspoon paprika

¼ teaspoon freshly ground black pepper

2 lemons, thinly sliced

1 small bunch assorted fresh herbs

3 garlic cloves

2 anchovies

1 head broccoli, cut into florets

Preheat the oven to 400°F.

Rub the trout generously with 1 tablespoon of the olive oil and sprinkle with the salt, paprika, and pepper. Place a quarter of the lemon slices and herbs in the cavity of each trout.

Set out four 8 × 8-inch sheets of parchment paper or aluminum foil on the countertop. Fold the edges of the parchment over the fish and secure with toothpicks or pinch the edges of the aluminum foil shut. Place on a baking sheet and transfer to the preheated oven. Bake for 20 to 25 minutes until the fish flakes when pressed with a fork and is cooked through.

Place the remaining 3 tablespoons olive oil, the garlic, and anchovies in a mini chopper or food processor and chop. Transfer to a large bowl along with the broccoli florets and toss well. Place the broccoli in another sheet of parchment paper or aluminum foil. Place on a separate baking sheet and transfer to the oven. Bake for 15 to 20 minutes until tender. Serve immediately with the fish.

NUTRITIONAL STATS PER SERVING (1 WHOLE TROUT WITH 1 CUP BROCCOLI): 327 Calories ❖ 26g Protein ❖ 9g Carbohydrates ❖ 21g Fat (3g Saturated) ❖ 68mg Cholesterol ❖ 2g Sugars ❖ 3g Fiber ❖ 430mg Sodium

Vitamin B_{12} = 213% ❖ Vitamin C = 140% ❖ DHA+EPA = 140% ❖ Vitamin K = 110% ❖ Vitamin A = 73%

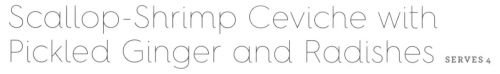
Scallop-Shrimp Ceviche with Pickled Ginger and Radishes SERVES 4

Ceviche makes for a fast, no-cook seafood dish that's ideal for a fresh summer meal. A staple of Mediterranean diets, this is a simple way to increase your seafood intake. It may be intimidating for seafood newbies, but it's actually quite easy, as the acid in the lime juice cooks the seafood. Another perk is that this dish does not leave your kitchen smelling like seafood. Shrimp and scallops bring you natural iodine and vitamin B_{12}, both of which keep your thyroid healthy. Shop for tangy pickled ginger in Asian grocery stores or opt for thinly sliced fresh ginger in its place. Reserve the pickled ginger from your next sushi order to use here.

½ pound sea scallops, diced

½ pound shrimp, cut into 1-inch-wide chunks

Juice of 4 limes

2 tomatoes, chopped

4 radishes, trimmed and thinly sliced

½ cup thinly sliced sweet white or red onion

2 tablespoons pickled ginger

1 tablespoon hot sauce (optional)

2 avocados, pitted, peeled, and cubed

16 large romaine leaves (about 2 heads)

Place the scallops, shrimp, lime juice, tomatoes, radishes, white or red onion, pickled ginger, and hot sauce, if using, in a large bowl. Toss well and cover with plastic wrap. Refrigerate for 15 to 20 minutes until the scallops and shrimp are firm to the touch and no longer translucent. Stir in the avocados. Set out the 16 romaine leaves and top each with 3 heaping tablespoons of the ceviche. Serve immediately.

NUTRITIONAL STATS PER SERVING (4 CEVICHE-FILLED LETTUCE LEAVES): 329 Calories ❖ 23g Protein ❖ 24g Carbohydrates ❖ 17g Fat (3g Saturated) ❖ 85mg Cholesterol ❖ 8g Sugars ❖ 12g Fiber ❖ 420mg Sodium

Vitamin K = 312% ❖ Vitamin C = 72% ❖ Iodine = 60% ❖ Vitamin B_{12} = 58% ❖ Fiber = 48%

Paprika Shrimp with Peppadew Peppers and Carrot-Sweet Potato Puree SERVES 4

Carrots blended with sweet potatoes make a solid foundation for spicy pickled peppadew peppers. To plan ahead for a party, make the puree the day before and store it in the fridge. You can gently rewarm it or serve it chilled. This puree also makes an excellent base for cooked fish.

1 red onion, peeled and thinly sliced

2 tablespoons raw apple cider vinegar

1 tablespoon olive oil

1 pound carrots, peeled and chopped

2 sweet potatoes, peeled and chopped

1 cup buttermilk

¼ teaspoon garlic salt

1 pound raw shrimp, peeled and deveined

½ teaspoon paprika

¼ teaspoon freshly ground black pepper

1 tablespoon olive oil

¼ cup peppadew peppers, chopped

Finely grated zest and juice of 1 lemon

Combine the red onion, apple cider vinegar, and olive oil in a medium bowl and toss well. Set aside.

Put the carrots and the sweet potatoes in a large saucepan, cover with cold water, and bring to a boil over high heat. Cover, reduce to a simmer, and cook for 8 to 10 minutes until the carrots and potatoes are tender. Drain and transfer to a food processor. Process until a chunky mixture forms. Add the buttermilk and garlic salt and process until smooth and creamy.

Sprinkle the shrimp with the paprika and the black pepper. Heat the olive oil a large skillet over high heat for 1 minute and then add the shrimp. Cook for 3 to 4 minutes, tossing, until the shrimp are pink and cooked through. Turn the heat off and stir in the peppadew peppers, lemon zest, and lemon juice.

Divide the puree among four plates and top with the shrimp mixture. Garnish each with a quarter of the reserved red onion.

NUTRITIONAL STATS PER SERVING (¼ POUND SHRIMP WITH PEPPADEWS, 1½ CUPS PUREE, AND GARNISH) 332 CALORIES ✦ **27g Protein** ✦ **35g Carbohydrates** ✦ **10g Fat (1g Saturated)** ✦ **145mg Cholesterol** ✦ **14g Sugars** ✦ **7g Fiber** ✦ **425mg Sodium**

Vitamin A = 212% ✦ Selenium = 65% ✦ Vitamin B$_{12}$ = 58% ✦ Vitamin C = 57% ✦ Protein = 59%

Grilled Oyster Tacos with Chipotle-Tomato Salsa SERVES 4

Oysters top my list of best brain foods because you get the hardest-to-find brain nutrients for just 10 to 20 calories per oyster: EPA+DHA, zinc, iron, iodine, and vitamin D. For those new to oysters, this is a nice option to try. Smoky chipotle salsa will have you hooked on this tempting and healthy meal. Find canned chipotle chiles in the Latin aisle.

4 unpeeled garlic cloves

1 small unpeeled onion

4 tomatoes (about 1 pound), quartered

Finely grated zest and juice of 1 lime

2 tablespoons olive oil

2 tablespoons chopped canned chipotle chiles in adobo sauce

½ teaspoon salt

2 dozen small to medium oysters, such as Blue Point

8 gluten-free corn tortillas, warmed on the grill

½ pound watercress

Preheat a grill over high heat.

Wrap the garlic cloves in a piece of aluminum foil and place on the grill along with the unwrapped onion. Grill for 3 to 4 minutes, until the garlic softens and the onion starts to brown. Transfer the onion and garlic to a cutting board to cool slightly.

When cool enough to handle, remove the skin from both and place in a food processor. Pulse 8 to 10 times until roughly chopped. Add the tomatoes, lime zest and juice, olive oil, chipotle chiles, and salt. Pulse again 5 to 6 times until a chunky salsa forms.

Place the oysters, flat side up, on the grill rack. Close the lid and grill until the top shells pop open, 3 to 5 minutes. Using tongs, transfer the oysters to the cutting

board; keep them level so the oyster "liquor" (salty seawater) doesn't spill out.

Wear an oven mitt to hold the oyster, and use a shucker to remove the top shell, cutting the oyster away from it and leaving it in the bottom shell. Set out the tortillas and top with a few sprigs of watercress, then spoon 3 oysters over each tortilla along with their juices. Top with 2 tablespoons of the salsa and serve immediately.

NUTRITIONAL STATS PER SERVING (2 CORN TORTILLAS, EACH WITH 3 OYSTERS): 313 Calories ❖ 20g Protein ❖ 34g Carbohydrates ❖ 11g Fat (2g Saturated) ❖ 85mg Cholesterol ❖ 4g Sugars ❖ 5g Fiber ❖ 230mg Sodium

Zinc = 570% ❖ Vitamin B$_{12}$ = 413% ❖ Vitamin C = 68% ❖ DHA+EPA = 68% ❖ Selenium = 49%

Crispy Arctic Char with Buttered Cauliflower SERVES 4

Dusting fish with oat flour and spices makes for a thin crispy crust without heavy breading or batter. Keep the heat at medium when cooking the fish to avoid burning the spices and causing the oil to smoke. For fish-and-chips lovers, serve malt vinegar on the side.

2 tablespoons olive oil

1 small head cauliflower, cut into florets

2 tablespoons unsalted grass-fed butter

½ teaspoon reduced-sodium Old Bay seasoning or grilling spices

¼ cup peppadew peppers, minced

4 arctic char fillets, skin on (about 16 ounces total)

1 teaspoon paprika

½ teaspoon garlic salt

¼ teaspoon freshly ground black pepper

½ cup oat flour

2 tablespoons coconut oil

Coat a large stockpot with a layer of olive oil and place over medium heat. Add the florets, cover, and cook for 4 to 5 minutes until the cauliflower starts to brown. Add the butter and continue to cook 1 minute, tossing well, until the cauliflower is well coated. Sprinkle with the Old Bay or other seasoning and the peppadew peppers, then turn off the heat.

Sprinkle the fish with the paprika, garlic salt, and black pepper. Place the oat flour on a plate and press both sides of the fish into the flour. Coat a large skillet with coconut oil and warm over medium heat. Add the fish, skin side down, and cook for 2 to 3 minutes, without moving it. Turn and cook for 2 minutes more.

Serve the fish immediately with the cauliflower.

NUTRITIONAL STATS PER SERVING (1 ARCTIC CHAR FILLET AND 1½ CUPS CAULIFLOWER): 412 Calories ❖ 29g Protein ❖ 21g Carbohydrates ❖ 20g Fat (7g Saturated) ❖ 47mg Cholesterol ❖ 3g Sugars ❖ 5g Fiber ❖ 266mg Sodium

Vitamin C = 96% ❖ Protein = 63% ❖ Vitamin K = 28% ❖ Folate = 25% ❖ Fiber = 20%

Baked Flaxseed Crab Cakes over Romaine Salad SERVES 4

You don't have to book a reservation at your favorite seafood house to dig into flaky crab cakes—just make these simple ones in your broiler at home! Crab is an overlooked superfood, low in calories and high in complete protein, vitamin B_{12}, and zinc, all key building blocks of your body and brain. Flaxseeds and hemp seeds bring in fiber and protein, so you stay full longer. If you spy reddish microgreens or fresh nasturtiums at your local farmers' market, they will make lovely garnishes for this gourmet meal and add a spicy note.

Olive oil cooking spray
1 pound lump crabmeat
4 scallions, chopped
2 tablespoons fresh hebs such as dill, chives, or tarragon

½ cup olive oil–based mayonnaise
¼ cup ground flaxseeds
¼ cup quick-cooking rolled oats
2 tablespoons hemp seeds

½ teaspoon seafood seasoning such as reduced-sodium Old Bay
½ pound romaine lettuce
1 tablespoon olive oil
1 tablespoon red wine vinegar

Position a rack in the center of the oven. Coat a baking sheet with olive oil cooking spray.

Pick through the crabmeat to make sure there aren't any shells. Set aside.

Put the scallions, fresh herbs, mayonnaise, and flaxseeds in a large bowl and stir well to combine. Add the crabmeat and give it a gentle toss.

Place the oats, hemp seeds, and seafood seasoning on a plate. Toss with your fingers to mix.

Form the crabmeat mixture into four 4-inch-wide patties and press into the oat-seed mixture. Transfer to the prepared baking sheet. Mist the tops with olive oil

cooking spray and transfer to the oven. Broil for 3 to 5 minutes until the tops are golden.

Place the romaine in a large bowl along with the olive oil and the vinegar and toss well. Divide the romaine salad among four plates. Top each plate with two crab cakes and serve immediately.

NUTRITIONAL STATS PER SERVING (1 CRAB CAKES WITH SALAD): 337 Calories ❖ 25g Protein ❖ 11g Carbohydrates ❖ 20g Fat (2g Saturated) ❖ 98mg Cholesterol ❖ 2g Sugars ❖ 4g Fiber ❖ 664mg Sodium

Vitamin B_{12} = 417% ❖ ALA = 155% ❖ Vitamin K = 83% ❖ DHA+EPA = 80% ❖ Protein = 54%

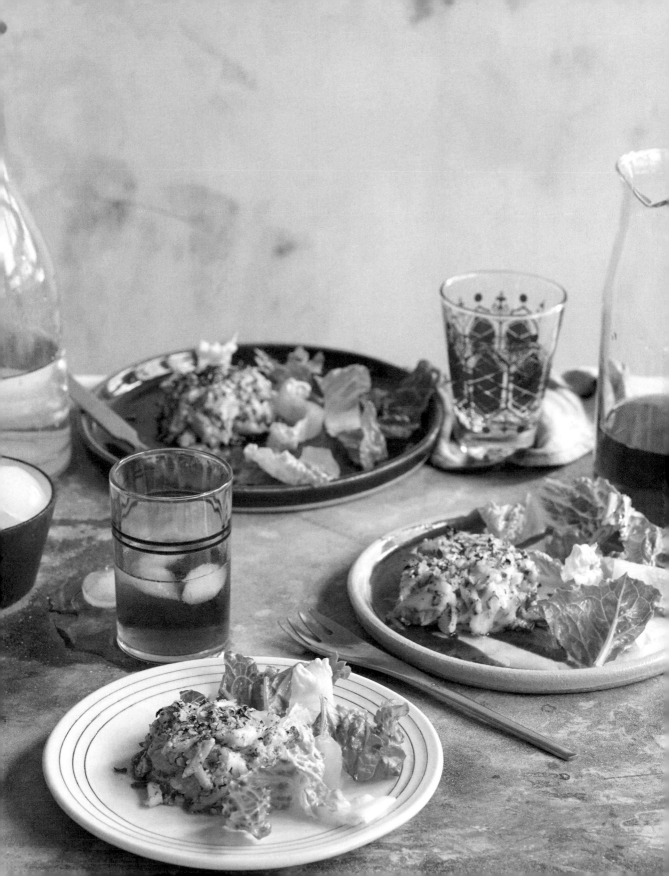

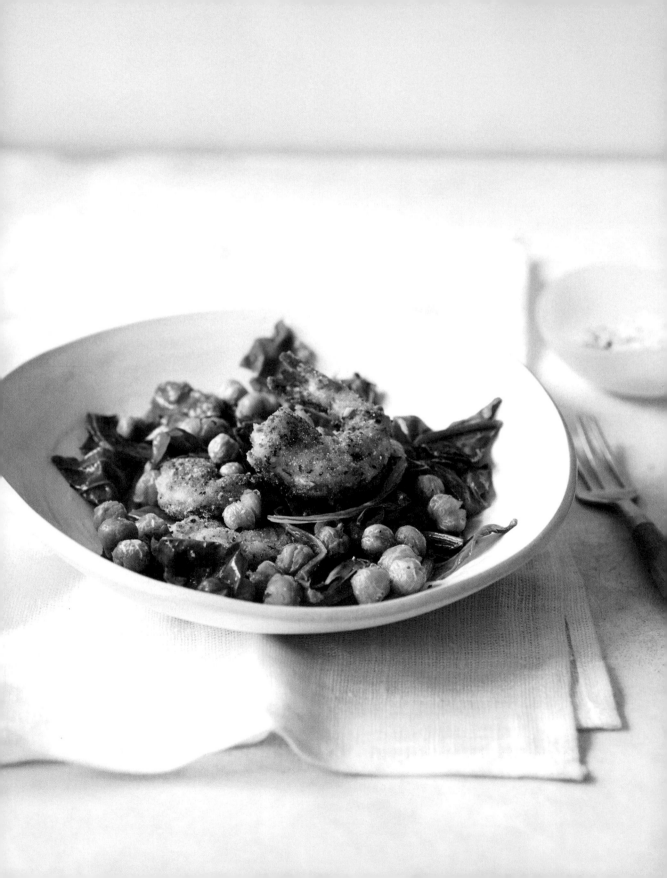

Crispy Shrimp with Greens and Beans SERVES 4

Lovers of fried seafood take note. This crispy panfry is a healthier option than your usual deep fry. Pick your shrimp well (wild with no salt preservative) for a high-protein, iodine-rich seafood option that is appealing for kids and those new to seafood. By subbing in the greens and beans for biscuits or fries, not only do you get a major nutrition boost, but you also load up on filling fiber.

½ cup gluten-free pancake mix

½ cup Parmesan cheese

2 tablespoons ground flaxseeds

2 tablespoons pumpkin seeds

1 teaspoon dried herbs, such as Italian seasoning

1 pasture-raised egg

1 pound large shrimp, peeled, deveined, tails removed

3 tablespoons olive oil

½ pound Swiss chard or kale, chopped

2 garlic cloves, thinly sliced

One 15.5-ounce can no-salt-added chickpeas or navy beans, rinsed well under cold running water and drained

Place the pancake mix, cheese, flaxseeds, pumpkin seeds, and herbs on a plate and toss with your fingers to mix.

Whisk the egg in a shallow bowl.

Dip a shrimp in the beaten egg and press into the pancake mixture, then transfer to a large clean plate. Repeat with the remaining shrimp, working in batches as needed, and place in the fridge while you prepare the greens.

Warm 1 tablespoon of the olive oil in a large skillet and add the greens and garlic. Toss well and cook for 1 to 2 minutes until the greens have wilted. Add the beans and toss again. Turn off the heat and set aside.

Heat a separate large skillet over medium heat and add the remaining 2 tablespoons olive oil. Add the shrimp and cook for 4 to 6 minutes, turning occasionally, until the shrimp are crispy and cooked through. Transfer to a plate lined with a paper towel.

Place the greens on four plates, dividing them equally, and top with the shrimp. Serve immediately.

NUTRITIONAL STATS PER SERVING (¼ POUND GREENS AND BEANS WITH 6 BREADED SHRIMP):
525 Calories ❖ 38g Protein ❖ 51g Carbohydrates ❖ 19g Fat (3g Saturated) ❖ 220mg Cholesterol ❖ 1g Sugars ❖ 11g Fiber ❖ 461mg Sodium

ALA = 128% ❖ Vitamin C = 125% ❖ Protein = 83% ❖ Selenium = 78% ❖ Folate = 40%

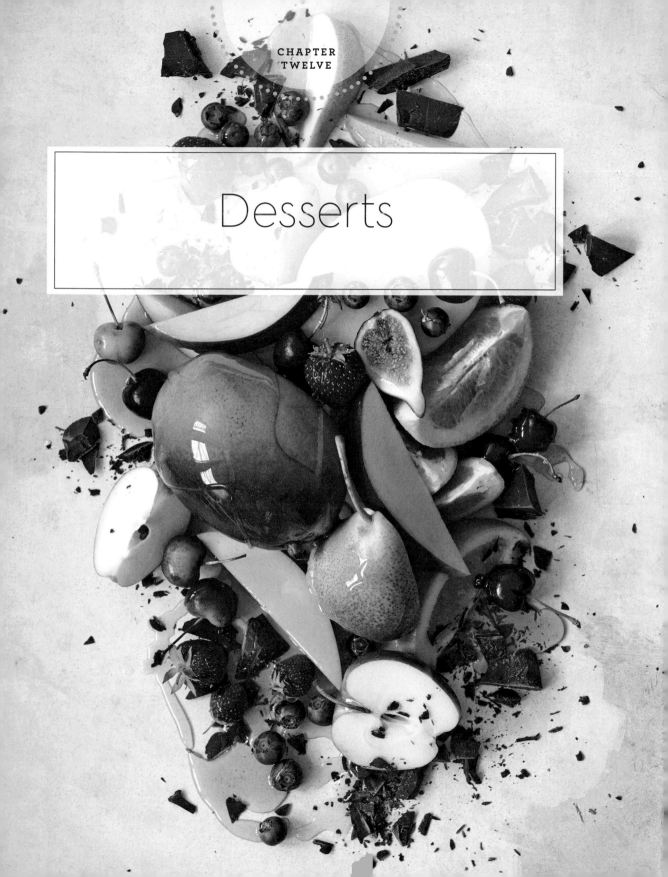

Desserts

Toasted Butter Pecan Kefir Sherbet SERVES 8

Looking for a frozen treat with health benefits? Kefir is a low-lactose, high-protein, fermented dairy product that contains the goodness of over ten probiotic cultures. Freezing it doesn't harm the cultures, but does give it a creamy ice cream–like texture. Good bugs, like the ones in kefir, help keep the microbiome healthy, which in turn affects your brain health. Egg yolks make this a dessert rich in choline, B vitamins, and vitamin D. This sherbet is a sweet, guilt-free choice when it comes to dessert.

4 cups light coconut milk

4 cups plain kefir

4 egg yolks, preferably from pasture-raised eggs

2 tablespoons unsalted grass-fed butter, at room temperature

¼ cup pure maple syrup

½ cup chopped toasted pecans

1 teaspoon pure vanilla extract

Place the coconut milk, kefir, egg yolks, butter, maple syrup, pecans, and vanilla in a blender and blend until smooth.

Pour the mixture into an ice cream maker and process according to the manufacturer's instructions.

Serve immediately after churning, or transfer to an airtight container and freeze until ready to serve.

NUTRITIONAL STATS PER SERVING (1 CUP): 227
Calories ❖ 7g Protein ❖ 18g Carbohydrates ❖ 14g Fat (8g Saturated) ❖ 3mg Cholesterol ❖ 14g Sugars ❖ 2g Fiber ❖ 73mg Sodium

Vitamin D = 27% ❖ Choline = 17% ❖ Calcium & Protein = 15% ❖ Vitamin A, Vitamin B$_{12}$ = 12% ❖ Iodine = 9%

Toasted Butter Pecan Kefir Sherbet;
Lemon Balm–Berry Sorbet

Lemon Balm–Berry Sorbet SERVES 8

Refresh yourself with this light yet luscious sorbet that is high in vitamin C. Lemon balm gives the sorbet a hint of citrus, but if you can't find this unique herb, flavor it with fresh mint or 1 tablespoon of finely grated lemon or grapefruit zest instead. Sorbets based on fruits and berries can deliver powerful flavors in small quantities. When you worry about indulging in dessert, think about this sorbet's high concentrations of flavonoids that help your body battle inflammation and aging.

1 quart fresh strawberries or 4 cups frozen strawberries

1 quart fresh blueberries or 4 cups frozen blueberries

2 cups seltzer water

¼ cup fresh lemon juice (about 1 lemon)

½ cup chopped fresh lemon balm leaves

1 tablespoon honey

Put the strawberries, blueberries, seltzer water, lemon juice, lemon balm, and honey in a blender. Blend until the berries are broken up and the mixture is fairly smooth.

Chill the mixture thoroughly, then freeze it in your ice cream maker according to the manufacturer's instructions. Serve immediately, or transfer to an airtight container and freeze until ready to serve.

NUTRITIONAL STATS PER SERVING (1 CUP): 82
Calories ❖ 1g Protein ❖ 20g Carbohydrates ❖ 0g Fat (0g Saturated) ❖ 0mg Cholesterol ❖ 15g Sugars ❖ 3g Fiber ❖ 2mg Sodium

Vitamin C = 71% ❖ Vitamin K = 30% ❖ Fiber = 12% ❖ Folate = 6% ❖ Thiamine, Magnesium = 5%

Double Chocolate–Avocado Mousse SERVES 4

This recipe for an avocado-based mousse blends the trifecta of dark chocolate, raspberries, and hemp. This indulgent mousse is both naughty and nice. On the naughty side, it tastes like the real McCoy, and not even the most devoted chocoholic will notice the avocado. On the nice side, it's great for your health—the avocado, dark chocolate (70% cocoa), and raspberries are all high in flavanols, and the hemp seeds provide you with manganese and magnesium.

½ cup chopped dark chocolate (70% cocoa)

⅓ cup grass-fed whole milk

3 tablespoons brown sugar

2 tablespoons unsweetened cocoa powder

2 teaspoons pure vanilla extract

2 avocados, pitted, peeled, and diced

1 cup raspberries

4 tablespoons hemp seeds

Place the chocolate, milk, sugar, cocoa powder, and vanilla in a small saucepan over medium heat. Stir until the chocolate is melted and smooth, about 3 minutes. Set aside to cool slightly.

Put the melted chocolate mixture and the avocados in the bowl of a food processor and blend until smooth and creamy, scraping down the sides of the bowl as needed. Spoon the mousse into glasses, sprinkle with raspberries and hemp seeds, cover with plastic wrap, and refrigerate for at least 3 hours.

NUTRITIONAL STATS PER SERVING (½ CUP): 309
Calories ❖ 5g Protein ❖ 29g Carbohydrates ❖ 19g Fat (8g Saturated) ❖ 3mg Cholesterol ❖ 20g Sugars ❖ 9g Fiber ❖ 20mg Sodium

Magnesium = 36% ❖ Fiber = 36% ❖ Iron = 26% ❖ Zinc = 24% ❖ Choline = 17%

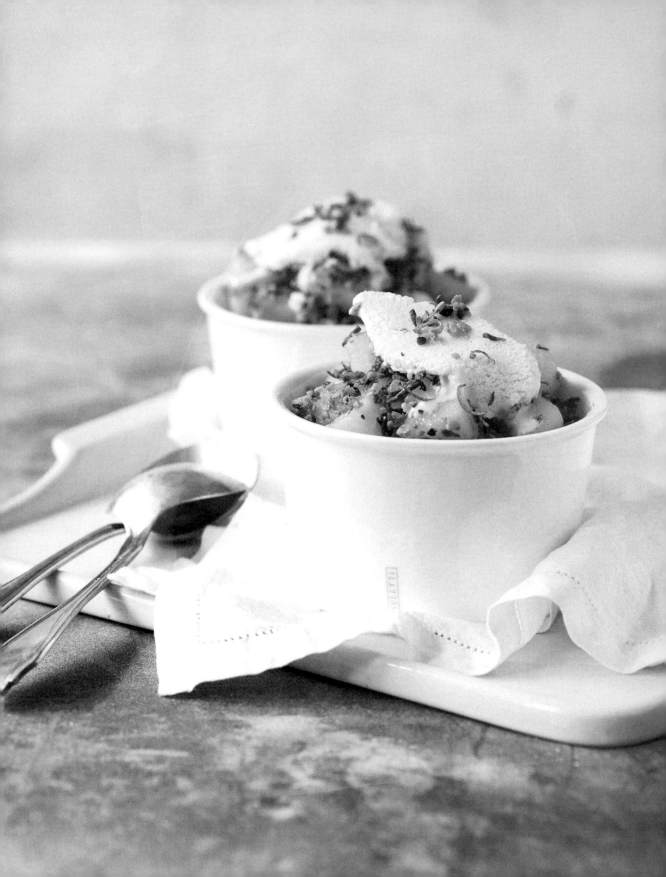

Turmeric-Mango Gratin SERVES 4

This high-fiber gratin is a treat of phytonutrients, and it can be whipped up in 10 minutes flat. Fusing sweet mellow mango with spicy black pepper and crunchy sweet coconut with a stringent turmeric, this gourmet dish is a molecular manifesto of brain health. From the rejuvenating curcumin in the turmeric to the soothing breeze of the liminoids in the lime zest, this dessert is doctor approved.

2 large ripe mangos
Finely grated zest and juice of 1 lime
¼ cup quick-cooking rolled oats

¼ cup hemp seeds
¼ cup unsweetened coconut
¼ teaspoon turmeric
⅛ teaspoon freshly ground black pepper

4 teaspoons unsalted grass-fed butter
1 cup plain kefir or butter pecan ice cream

Position a rack in the middle of the oven. Preheat the broiler.

Using a heavy, sharp knife, slice the mangos lengthwise around each side of the pit. Remove the skin and cut the fruit into bite-size pieces. Transfer to a large bowl along with the lime zest and juice and toss well.

Put the oats, hemp seeds, coconut, turmeric, and black pepper in a small bowl and toss well to combine.

Place four ramekins on a baking sheet. Divide the mango mixture equally among the four ramekins. Sprinkle the oat mixture over each ramekin. Top each with 1 teaspoon of butter.

Transfer the baking sheet to the oven and broil the gratins for 2 to 3 minutes, or just until the topping has melted and browned. Serve immediately topped with ¼ cup kefir or butter pecan ice cream.

NUTRITIONAL STATS PER SERVING (1 GRATIN WITH KEFIR): 204 Calories ❖ 6g Protein ❖ 22g Carbohydrates ❖ 0g Fat (4g Saturated) ❖ 11mg Cholesterol ❖ 15g Sugars ❖ 3g Fiber ❖ 18mg Sodium

Vitamin C = 53% ❖ Magnesium = 27% ❖ Zinc = 16% ❖ Vitamin A = 15% ❖ Protein = 13%

Chocolate-Spiced Truffles MAKES 32 TRUFFLES

A nutrient-dense chocolate truffle? You don't have to be a professional pastry chef to make these delectable yet simple truffles that also happen to be high in vitamin E and fiber. Make them to wow your sweetheart, as a rainy-day project with the kids, or to tame the wild chocoholic in your life. Molecules found in cacao appear to reverse age-related memory decline, so you will be sure to remember these after eating them.

1 cup almonds
¼ cup pumpkin seeds
½ cup heavy cream

½ teaspoon ground cinnamon
¼ teaspoon ground cloves
⅛ teaspoon ground coriander

8 ounces bittersweet chocolate (70% cocoa), finely chopped
2 tablespoons unsweetened cocoa powder

Line a baking sheet with parchment or wax paper.

Put the almonds and pumpkin seeds in a food processor and finely chop.

In a small saucepan over medium-high heat, bring the cream, cinnamon, cloves, and coriander to a boil. Add the chocolate and let sit for 2 to 3 minutes, then whisk until smooth.

Stir in the almond–pumpkin seed mix. Cool to room temperature, then refrigerate, uncovered, until the mixture is firm, about 1 hour.

Spoon mounds (1 heaping teaspoonful each) of chocolate mixture onto the lined baking sheet. Return to the refrigerator for 15 minutes.

Roll the mounds into even smooth balls. Put the cocoa powder on a plate. Roll the balls in cocoa, and transfer the truffles to a small tray. Chill until set, about 30 minutes. Serve immediately or store, refrigerated, in an airtight container for up to 2 weeks.

NUTRITIONAL STATS PER SERVING (2 TRUFFLES):
146 Calories ❖ 3g Protein ❖ 9g Carbohydrates ❖ 13g Fat (5g Saturated) ❖ 10mg Cholesterol ❖ 4g Sugars ❖ 2g Fiber ❖ 3mg Sodium

Magnesium = 11% ❖ Fiber = 8% ❖ Protein = 7% ❖ Zinc, Iron = 6% ❖ Vitamin A = 4%

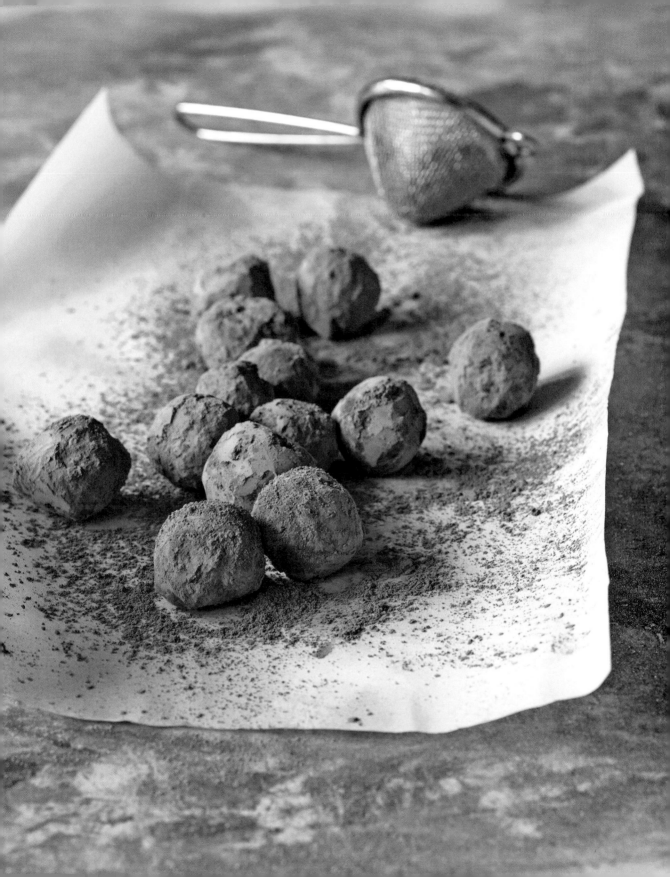

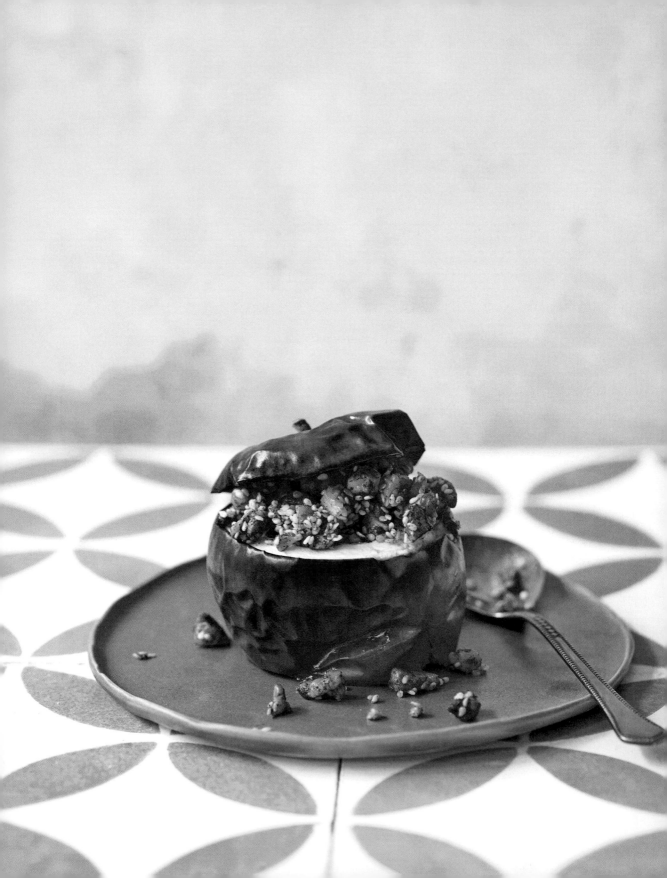

Sesame Seed–Cinnamon Baked Apples SERVES 4

Comforting baked apples are the ideal fall or winter treat. Soothe yourself in the chilly months when work schedules and school days can leave you feeling spent. Make a double batch of these apples on the weekend to warm up during the week, or add the leftovers to a morning smoothie made with kefir and sunflower seeds or nut butter.

4 apples, cored and seeded
¼ cup finely chopped walnuts
2 tablespoons sesame seeds

4 teaspoons olive oil or coconut oil
1 teaspoon ground cinnamon

1 teaspoon pure vanilla extract
¼ teaspoon ground turmeric

Preheat the oven to 350°F.

Place the apples in an 8 × 8-inch baking dish. Put the walnuts, sesame seeds, oil, cinnamon, vanilla, and turmeric in a small bowl and stir well with a teaspoon. Spoon the mixture into the cavity of each apple.

Bake the apples, uncovered, for 50 to 60 minutes until they puff and start to break apart. Let cool for 5 minutes before serving.

NUTRITIONAL STATS PER SERVING (1 BAKED APPLE): 212 Calories ❖ 2g Protein ❖ 27g Carbohydrates ❖ 11g Fat (1g Saturated) ❖ 0mg Cholesterol ❖ 19g Sugars ❖ 5g Fiber ❖ 2mg Sodium

Fiber = 20% ❖ Vitamin A = 15% ❖ Magnesium = 12% ❖ Vitamin C = 11% ❖ Vitamin E = 10%

Cashew-Banana Bread SERVES 10

If you don't tell them, they will never know: this bread is gluten-free, but oh so good! It may seem slightly underbaked when removed from the oven, but the thirsty coconut will absorb the moisture and firm its texture as it cools. To keep the bread from drying out, wrap it in a sheet of wax paper followed by a sheet of aluminum foil once it has cooled.

Olive oil, for greasing the pan
½ cup packed brown sugar
2 tablespoons coconut oil
2 large and very ripe bananas, mashed

1 pasture-raised egg
¾ cup gluten-free pancake mix
½ cup unsweetened shredded coconut
½ cup ground almonds

1 teaspoon baking powder
1 teaspoon ground cinnamon
¼ cup chopped cashews or macadamia nuts

Preheat the oven to 350°F. Coat a 2-pound loaf pan with olive oil.

In a mixing bowl, beat the brown sugar and coconut oil with an electric mixer fitted with the paddle on high speed until smooth and creamy, about 1 minute. Add the bananas and egg and mix again for 30 seconds until combined. Add the pancake mix, coconut, almonds, baking powder, and cinnamon and beat on low speed for 1 minute until well combined. Transfer the batter to the prepared loaf pan and sprinkle the top with the cashews or macadamia nuts.

Bake for 40 to 50 minutes until the edges start to brown and the center is firm to the touch. Cool in the pan for 5 minutes, then turn out of the pan and cool on a rack.

Slice the loaf into 10 portions and serve, or store in an airtight container on the countertop for up to 5 days.

NUTRITIONAL STATS PER SERVING (ONE 2-OZ SLICE): 185 Calories ❖ 2g Protein ❖ 26g Carbohydrates ❖ 8g Fat (4g Saturated) ❖ 0mg Cholesterol ❖ 10g Sugars ❖ 2g Fiber ❖ 91mg Sodium

Vitamin E = 12% ❖ Magnesium = 10% ❖ Fiber = 8% ❖ Zinc, Thiamine = 5% ❖ Calcium = 4% ❖ Protein = 4%

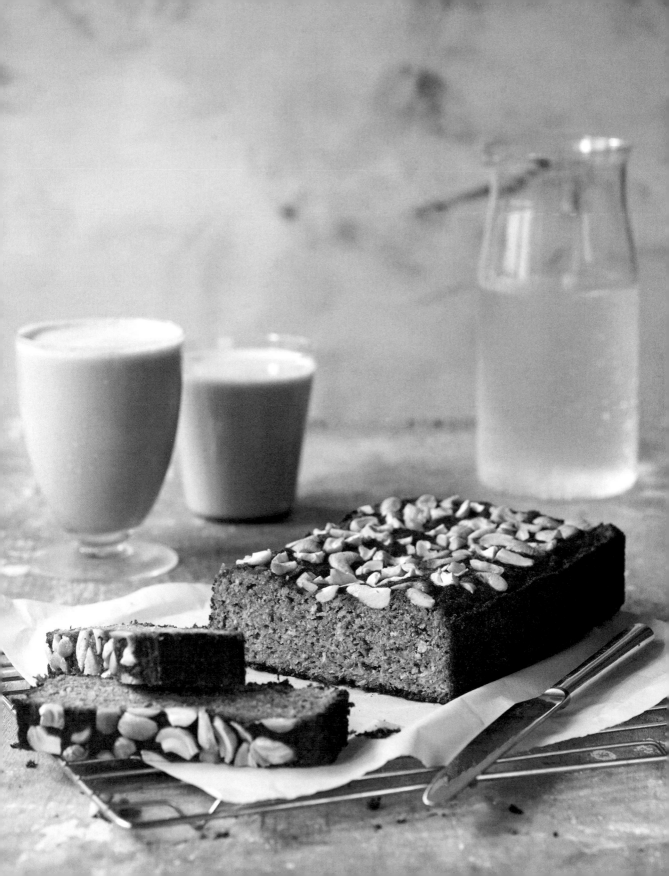

Cinnamon-Almond Egg Cream SERVES 2

The history of this eggless drink is foggy, but some say that the theater pioneer Boris Thomashevsky wanted to imitate a French drink called *chocolat et crème,* and it got lost in translation, coming out as "egg cream" instead. Regardless, this refreshing soda drink still soothes a sweet tooth, and its frothy top makes you think of whipped eggs.

1 cup grass-fed whole milk
2 teaspoons honey

½ teaspoon ground cinnamon
¼ teaspoon pure almond extract

1 cup seltzer
1 teaspoon unsweetened cocoa powder

Put the milk, honey, cinnamon, and almond extract in a pitcher and stir well. Divide the mixture between two glasses. Top with the seltzer and sprinkle with the cocoa powder. Serve immediately.

NUTRITIONAL STATS PER SERVING (1 CUP): 117
Calories ❖ 4g Protein ❖ 16g Carbohydrates ❖ 4g Fat (2g Saturated) ❖ 12mg Cholesterol ❖ 12g Sugars ❖ 0g Fiber ❖ 52mg Sodium

Vitamin D = 16% ❖ Calcium = 15% ❖ Vitamin B$_{12}$ = 9% ❖ Selenium = 7% ❖ Zinc and Magnesium = 4%

Turmeric-Cinnamon Macaroon MAKES 2 DOZEN

The taste of almond in these heavenly macaroons blends with the turmeric, creating a smooth but exotic flavor. After a few bites, you may get a bit of heat from the black pepper, but it won't keep you from going back for seconds! Instead, it will ensure that you reap the benefits of the turmeric, as pepper boosts the absorption of its healing properties by 2,000 percent.

1 cup unsweetened coconut
1 cup finely ground almonds
1 teaspoon ground cinnamon
¼ teaspoon ground turmeric

⅛ teaspoon freshly ground black pepper
4 extra-large egg whites, preferably from pasture-raised eggs, at room temperature

¼ teaspoon salt
½ cup granulated sugar
1 teaspoon pure vanilla extract

Preheat the oven to 325°F. Line two 18 × 13-inch sheet pans with parchment paper.

Combine the coconut, almonds, cinnamon, turmeric, and pepper in a large bowl.

In the bowl of an electric mixer fitted with the whisk attachment, whip the egg whites and salt on high speed until they form medium-firm peaks and stick to the sides of the bowl when it is tilted. With the mixer running, add the sugar in a steady stream.

Carefully fold the egg whites mixture and vanilla into the coconut mixture with a rubber spatula. Using a soup spoon, drop heaping tablespoons of the batter onto the prepared sheet pans.

Bake the macaroons for 25 to 30 minutes until golden brown. Let cool for 5 minutes before serving, or cool completely before storing in an airtight container for up to 1 week.

NUTRITIONAL STATS PER SERVING (1 COOKIE):
55 Calories ❖ 2g Protein ❖ 3g Carbohydrates ❖ 4g Fat (1g Saturated) ❖ 31mg Cholesterol ❖ 2g Sugars ❖ 1g Fiber ❖ 36mg Sodium

Zinc, Selenium, Iron = 5% ❖ Magnesium, Protein, Fiber = 4% ❖ Vitamin D, Vitamin B$_{12}$ = 3% ❖ Calcium, Vitamin A, Folate = 2% ❖ Potassium, Thiamine = 1%

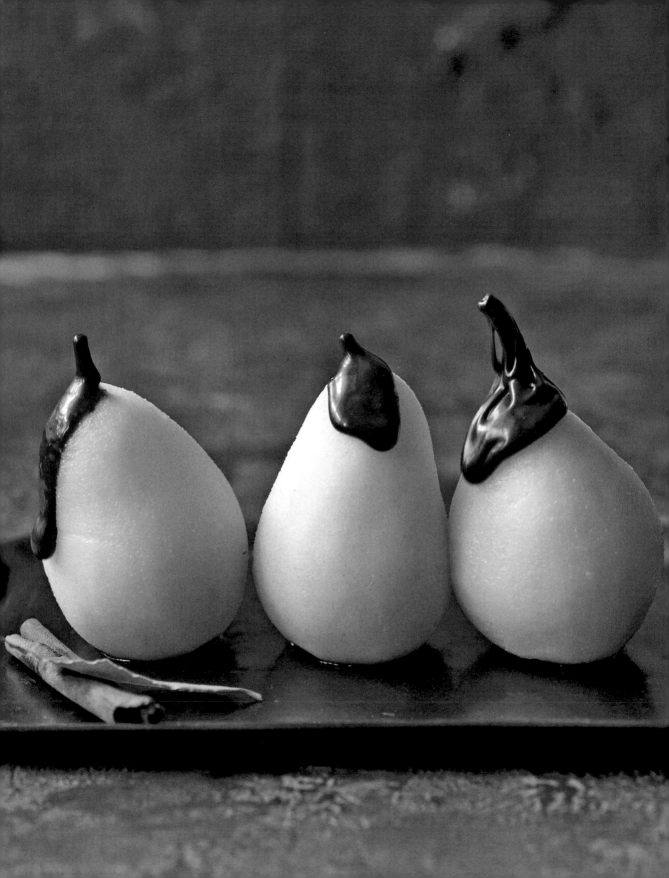

Nutmeg Poached Pears with Dark Fudge Sauce SERVES 4

Looking for a dessert with benefits? This one will fill you up at only 147 calories, since it packs 5 grams of fiber per serving. Remember that the darker the chocolate, the more cacao flavonoids there are in the sauce, and these flavonoids boost blood flow to the brain. Pair this hearty dessert with a lighter dinner or lunch, such as the Marinated Kale Salad (page 177) or another selection from the salad section.

4 pears, peeled and cored
1 cinnamon stick
2 bay leaves

1 tablespoon black peppercorns
½ teaspoon freshly grated nutmeg

4 tablespoons good-quality, store-bought dark chocolate fudge sauce

Place the pears, cinnamon stick, bay leaves, black peppercorns, and half the nutmeg in a large stockpot and cover with water. Bring to a boil over high heat. Turn off the heat and let cool to room temperature. Drain the pears, sprinkle with the remaining nutmeg, and top with the chocolate sauce.

NUTRITIONAL STATS PER SERVING (1 PEAR WITH 1 TABLESPOON CHOCOLATE SAUCE): 147 Calories ❖ 1g Protein ❖ 37g Carbohydrates ❖ 1g Fat (0g Saturated) ❖ 0mg Cholesterol ❖ 26g Sugars ❖ 5g Fiber ❖ 9mg Sodium

Fiber = 20% ❖ Vitamin C = 9% ❖ Vitamin K = 8% ❖ Potassium, Magnesium = 4% ❖ Folate = 3%

Calm the Storm
Sleep-Remedy Tea SERVES 4

This tasty caffeine-free tea contains three ingredients shown to soothe and calm. Naturally sweet-tasting mint has been proved to soothe digestion, and cardamom works as a carminative to prevent bloating. Saint-John's-Wort is a proven antidepressant and appears to work by calming the brain's stress response. (Regular use of Saint-John's-Wort without consulting a physician should be avoided, as it can interfere with some medications.)

4½ cups water
4 Saint-John's-Wort tea bags

1 cup fresh mint leaves

¼ teaspoon ground cardamom

Bring a large saucepan filled with the 4½ cups water to a boil. Add the tea bags and the mint and let steep for 3 to 4 minutes. Drain, sprinkle with cardamom, and serve.

NUTRITIONAL STATS PER SERVING (1 CUP):
5 Calories ✤ 0g Protein ✤ 1g Carbohydrates ✤ 0g Fat (0g Saturated) ✤ 0mg Cholesterol ✤ 0g Sugars ✤ 0g Fiber ✤ 2mg Sodium

2–3% of Vitamin C, Folate, Vitamin K, Calcium, Iron, Magnesium

Nutty Cacao Brain Bars MAKES 10 BARS

These fun no-bake bars are irresistibly crunchy thanks to the cracked cacao nibs. Bitter cacao nibs carry a host of nutrients and contrast nicely with the sweet dates and honey. Nibs provide more of the the flavonoids from the cacao, which are the phytonutirents known to improve brain function and possibly even reverse memory decline. Shop for high-quality cacao nibs in health food stores, and store them in the fridge to keep their vital fats from going rancid.

Olive oil
½ cup (packed) dates, pitted
1 cup rolled oats

½ cup roasted unsalted almonds, roughly chopped
½ cup sunflower seeds
¾ cup cacao nibs

½ cup creamy peanut butter or almond butter
¼ cup honey

Coat an 8 × 8-inch baking dish with olive oil.

Put the dates in a food processor and process until a thick paste forms. Add the oats and almonds and pulse until a chunky mixture forms and the dates are evenly distributed. Transfer the mixture to a large bowl. Stir in the sunflower seeds and the cacao nibs.

Combine the peanut butter or almond butter and the honey in a small saucepan over low heat and cook, stirring, until well mixed. Pour over the oat mixture and mix well with a wooden spoon until a thick and gooey paste forms.

Transfer the mixture to the prepared baking dish and press down with a rubber spatula to flatten. Cover with parchment paper or plastic wrap and transfer to the fridge or freezer for 15 to 20 minutes until set and hardened.

Remove from the baking dish and cut into 10 even bars. Store in an airtight container for up to 5 days.

NUTRITIONAL STATS PER SERVING (1 BAR):
230 Calories ❖ 6g Protein ❖ 27g Carbohydrates ❖ 12g Fat (4g Saturated) ❖ 0mg Cholesterol ❖ 14g Sugars ❖ 5g Fiber ❖ 30mg Sodium

Magnesium = 21% ❖ Fiber = 20% ❖ Vitamin E = 15% ❖ Protein = 12% ❖ Zinc = 10%

Mixed-Nut Cardamom Baklava Bites MAKES 20 PIECES

Try these sumptuous baklava bites, minus the phyllo, to get the same honeyed nut dessert without all the work. If you're a "frozen candy bar" fan, these will be your new, more nutrient-dense love. Just transfer them to an airtight container and place in the freezer for up to 6 months—if they survive snack attacks, that is!

1 cup Brazil nuts (about 4 ounces)

1 cup walnuts (about 4 ounces)

½ cup pumpkin seeds (about 2 ounces)

½ cup almonds (about 2 ounces)

1 teaspoon ground cinnamon

½ teaspoon ground cardamom

½ cup almond butter, at room temperature

6 tablespoons honey

¼ cup unsalted grass-fed butter, at room temperature

½ teaspoon pure vanilla extract

¼ teaspoon salt

Place the Brazil nuts in a food processor and pulse about 10 times until roughly chopped. Add the walnuts, pumpkin seeds, almonds, cinnamon, and cardamom and pulse another 10 times until the nuts and seeds are finely chopped. Transfer 1 cup of the chopped nuts to a plate to use as a coating later.

To the remaining nuts in the food processor, add the almond butter, 5 tablespoons of the honey, the butter, and vanilla and pulse 8 to 10 times more until a thick paste forms. Roll the mixture into balls about 1 inch in diameter until you have 20 bites. Then roll them in the reserved chopped nuts.

Just before serving, drizzle them with the remaining 1 tablespoon honey and sprinkle with the salt. Serve immediately or store in an airtight container on the countertop for up to 5 days.

NUTRITIONAL STATS PER SERVING (1 PIECE):
214 Calories ❖ 6g Protein ❖ 10g Carbohydrates ❖ 19g Fat (4g Saturated) ❖ 6mg Cholesterol ❖ 6g Sugars ❖ 2g Fiber ❖ 31mg Sodium

ALA = 239% ❖ Thiamine = 23% ❖ Vitamin E = 20% ❖ Magnesium = 16% ❖ Selenium = 15%

Flourless Chocolate-Almond Cake SERVES 10

This fudgy cake is sinfully good and has a surprising afternote of spicy cayenne. Almonds are the top source of the hard-to-find vitamin E, a brain-protecting champion that is woefully underconsumed. This cake is a great excuse to get more almonds in your diet. To fully elevate this dessert, serve it with ¼ cup of the Toasted Butter Pecan Kefir Sherbet (page 260).

Butter or olive oil, for baking dish

8 ounces bittersweet (at least 60% cocoa) chocolate, chopped

½ cup heavy cream, preferably from grass-fed cows

1 cup ground almonds

½ cup packed brown sugar

½ teaspoon baking soda

¼ teaspoon ground cayenne pepper

5 large pasture-raised eggs, separated

⅛ teaspoon salt

¼ cup unsweetened cocoa powder

Preheat oven to 350°F. Grease an 8 × 8-inch baking dish with butter or olive oil.

Place the chocolate and heavy cream in a large saucepan and set over medium-low heat. Cook for 1 to 2 minutes, stirring often, until the chocolate is melted and smooth. Remove from the heat and stir in the almonds, brown sugar, baking soda, and cayenne. Stir in the egg yolks and set aside.

Place the egg whites and salt in a large mixing bowl and beat with an attachment fitted with the whisk on high speed until the egg whites form soft peaks. Fold the egg whites into the chocolate mixture.

Transfer the batter to the prepared 8 × 8-inch baking dish. Bake until puffed and firm around the edges, 35 to 40 minutes for a soft cake and 50 to 55 minutes for a firmer cake.

Run a knife around the edge of the cake to loosen it, and then cut into 10 pieces. Dust with the cocoa powder and serve warm. Alternatively, let cool to room temperature and serve or chill 1 hour before serving.

NUTRITIONAL STATS PER SERVING (1 SLICE):
277 Calories ❖ 8g Protein ❖ 21g Carbohydrates ❖ 22g Fat (10g Saturated) ❖ 110mg Cholesterol ❖ 14g Sugars ❖ 4g Fiber ❖ 136mg Sodium

ALA = 150% ❖ Vitamin E = 30% ❖ Protein = 17% ❖ Fiber = 16% ❖ Selenium = 15%

Polka Dot Lemon Squares with Poppy Seeds SERVES 12

A tart but sweet lemon square is a true delight. This speckled version, at only 146 calories a bar, has a nutrition boost from the nuts, coconut, and seeds, all while scaling back on the amount of sugar used in a traditional recipe. These squares are a great way to get more nuts and seeds into your diet. Pumpkin seeds are rich in much-needed zinc and magnesium, both of which stimulate brain growth.

Crust
Olive oil
⅓ cup pumpkin seeds
¼ cup walnuts or almonds
½ cup unsweetened shredded coconut

1 tablespoon coconut oil
1 tablespoon cold water

Filling
4 large whole pasture-raised eggs, plus 2 egg yolks

¾ cup granulated sugar
1 teaspoon finely grated lemon zest
1 cup fresh lemon juice (about 8 lemons)
2 tablespoons poppy seeds

Position a rack in the middle of the oven and preheat the oven to 350°F. Grease an 8 × 8-inch baking pan with olive oil.

Make the crust: Put the pumpkin seeds and walnuts or almonds in the food processor and process until finely chopped. Add the coconut and process again until a fine meal forms. Add the coconut oil and cold water and pulse 3 to 4 times until a chunky mixture forms.

Press the nut mixture into the bottom of the prepared pan in an even layer. Bake for 10 to 15 minutes until firm to the touch. Remove from the oven and decrease the oven temperature to 300°F.

Meanwhile, make the filling: Whisk the whole eggs, egg yolks, sugar, lemon zest,

lemon juice, and poppy seeds in a large bowl until smooth. Pour the filling over the warm crust and return to the oven. Bake until the filling is just set, 30 to 35 minutes.

Let the bars cool in the pan on a rack, then refrigerate until firm, at least 2 hours. Cut into 12 squares and serve.

NUTRITIONAL STATS PER SERVING (1 SQUARE):
219 Calories ❖ 6g Protein ❖ 14g Carbohydrates ❖ 8g Fat (3g Saturated) ❖ 92mg Cholesterol ❖ 12g Sugars ❖ 1g Fiber ❖ 26mg Sodium

Selenium = 14% ❖ Protein = 13% ❖ Choline = 12% ❖ Vitamin C, Magnesium = 11% ❖ Zinc, Vitamin D = 10%

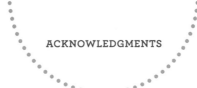

ACKNOWLEDGMENTS

This book was created with the encouragement and support of many: family, colleagues, and friends. E-mails, notes, and supportive comments from readers of my previous two books were a regular, surprising, and uplifting occurrence. Thank you.

My patients deserve special acknowledgment. I'm very grateful for your trust and quite honored to serve you. I appreciate the many ways you have all influenced my growth as a physician and helped me understand how to best prescribe food.

While the publishing world is rapidly changing, I've been blessed with the same team for all of my books: Karen Rinaldi and Julie Will, two stars of the publishing universe. Thank you for your friendship, guidance, and creativity. More authors need publishers like you. Sarah Murphy had the awful task of editing my first draft and holding me to deadlines, and she did this with consummate professionalism. Thank you. I'd be nowhere without Joy Tutela and the David Black Agency for making my proposals sing and getting my books published.

This book has delicious recipes because of the great creativity and skill of chef Jennifer Iserloh, coauthor of *50 Shades of Kale* and the culinary brain behind dozens of bestselling cookbooks. Thank you for another great project together and a fun collaboration. For the photographs, I was thrilled to work with another veteran professional of the food world, photographer Ellen Silverman, along with food stylist Eugene Jho, prop stylist Nidia Cueva, and their team. I am grateful for your wonderful eye, attention to detail, and immense work ethic.

My professional colleagues in psychiatry and mental health are all quick with a word of encouragement or a kale joke.

The New York State Psychiatric Institute and the Columbia University Department of Psychiatry have been my professional home since I moved to New York in 2000. I'm especially grateful to Lloyd Sederer and Deborah Cabaniss for leading the Columbia Psychiatry writing group, as well as the group members, all of whom actively write for the public. Philip Muskin has always made sure my eye is on the science. I'm grateful to our chairman, Jeffrey Lieberman, for his guidance over the years. Thank you to Sharon Akabas and Marie St. Onge at the Columbia University Institute of Human Nutrition (IHN) for the opportunity to serve as a thesis mentor and to teach. Cheers to the residents, to Eileen Kavanagh, and to the team at PIRC.

For the last four years, the American Psychiatric Association has featured our workshop, Food and the Brain, which I co-lead with two amazing psychiatrists, Emily Deans and Laura Lachance. Much of this book was validated by the research on the Brain Food Scale that was completed with Dr. Lachance and Ariel Suazo-Maler, my IHN graduate student. I'm inspired by my colleagues around the world who helped create the International Society of Nutrition and Psychiatry Research, and I'm especially grateful for the friendship and collaboration of Felice Jacka and Jerome Sarris.

Many thanks to my friends at the Center for Mind-Body Medicine, who serve up some of the most delicious medical education in the country at their trainings such as Food as Medicine and Mind-Body Medicine. Jim Gordon, Kathie Swift, and Mark Petus have been instrumental to my thinking about health, food, and self-care. Thank you to the big family at Eskenazi Health and Lisa Harris for showing us what can really be accomplished with health care.

The last few years have yielded relationships with some of the top movers and shakers in the wellness world. Thank you Mind, Body, Green, Well+Good NYC, the Brooklyn Grange, Wellness in the Schools, the *Huffington Post*, Even Hotels, Live Happy, Kripalu Center, and the New York Academy of Medicine.

The team at National Kale Day reminds me of the ways little ideas can grow. Many thanks to Uli and Jen Iserloh, Ellen Emerson, Melinda Goodwin, and Kristin Ziegelbauer for your inspiring work ethic and dedication. A vegetable never had it so good.

Finally, my friends and family have steadily supported me through the writing and publication of three books in the last five years. And what good times we have had together. Thanks for the care, friendship, and support. And thank you to New York City for all the great meals.

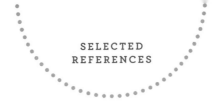

SELECTED
REFERENCES

The science supporting the impact of food on brain health is conclusive and compelling enough that I wrote this cookbook. Many subjects in nutrition are hotly debated, and I hope you will add your voice to the conversation. These references are a set of academic and research papers for a deeper dive into the science.

Two resources provide excellent overviews on nutrition and health. The first is the full text of the Food and Nutrition Board Dietary Reference Intakes for each nutrient, which can be found at https://fnic.nal.usda.gov/dietary-guidance/dietary-reference -intakes/dri-nutrient-reports. The second is the recently released 2015–2020 United States Department of Health and Human Services and Department of Agriculture's Dietary Guidelines for Americans, which can be found at http://health.gov/ dietaryguidelines/2015/guidelines/.

You can find full text versions for many of these articles on my website at Drew RamseyMD.com/studies.

Akbaraly, T. N., E. J. Brunner, J. E. Ferrie, M. G. Marmot, M. Kivimaki, and A. Singh-Manoux. "Dietary Pattern and Depressive Symptoms in Middle Age," *British Journal of Psychiatry* 195, no. 5 (Nov. 2009): 408–13.

Akkasheh, G., Z. Kashini-Poor, et al. "Clinical and metabolic response to probiotic administration in patients with major depressive disorder: A randomized, double-blind, placebo-controlled trial," *Nutrition* Sep 28 epub doi: 10.1016/j.nut.2015.09.003.

Amminger, G. P., M. R. Schäfer, K. Papageorgiou, S. M. Cotton, et al. "Long-chain omega-3 fatty acids for indicated prevention of psychotic disorders: a randomized, placebo-controlled trial," *Archives of General Psychiatry* 67, no. 2 (Feb. 2010): 146–54.

Baines, S., J. Powers, and W. J. Brown. "How does the health and wellbeing of young Australian vegetarian and semi-vegetarian women compare with non-vegetarians?" *Public Health Nutrition* 10, no. 5 (May 2007): 436–42.

Bantle, J. P. "Dietary fructose and metabolic syndrome and diabetes," *Journal of Nutrition* 139, no. 6 (June 2009): 1263S-8S.

Beezhold, B. L., C. S. Johnston, and D. R. Daigle. "Vegetarian diets are associated with healthy mood states: a cross-sectional study in seventh day Adventist adults," *Nutrition Journal* 1, no. 9 (June 2010): 26.

Bjelland, I., G. S. Tell, S. E. Vollset, S. Konstantinova, and P. M. Ueland. "Choline in anxiety and depression: the Hordaland Health Study," *American Journal of Clinical Nutrition* 90, no. 4 (Oct. 2009): 1056-60.

Brinkworth, G. D., J. D. Buckley, M. Noakes, P. M. Clifton, and C. J. Wilson. "Long-term effects of a very low-carbohydrate diet and a low-fat diet on mood and cognitive function," *Archives of Internal Medicine* 169, no. 20 (Nov. 2009): 1873-80.

Chowdhury, Rajiv, Samantha Warnakula, et al. "Association of dietary, circulating, and supplement fatty acids with coronary risk: a systemic review and meta-analysis," *Annals of Internal Medicine* 160, no. 6 (Mar. 2014): 398-406.

Conklin, S. M., P. J. Gianaros, S. M. Brown, J. K. Yao, A. R. Hariri, S. B. Manuck, and M. F. Muldoon. "Long-chain omega-3 fatty acid intake is associated positively with corticolimbic gray matter volume in healthy adults," *Neurosicence Letters* 421, no. 3 (June 2007): 209-12.

Crawford, M. A., C. L. Broadhurst, S. Cunnane, and D. E. Marsh. "Nutritional armor in evolution: docosahexaenoic acid as a determinant of neural, evolution and hominid brain development," *Military Medicine* 179, no. 11 Supplement (Nov. 2014): 61-75.

Daniel, C. R., A. J. Cross, C. Koebnick, and R. Sinha. "Trends in meat consumption in the United States," *Public Health Nutrition* 14, no. 4 (April 2011): 575-83.

Dror, D. K., and L. H. Allen. "Effect of vitamin B_{12} deficiency on neurodevelopment in infants: current knowledge and possible mechanisms," *Nutrition Reviews* 66, no. 5 (May 2008): 250-55.

Ervin, R. B. "Prevalence of metabolic syndrome among adults 20 years of age and over, by sex, age, race and ethnicity, and body mass index: United States 2003–2006," *National Health Statistics Reports* 13 (2009):1-8.

Fernandez, M. L. "Rethinking dietary cholesterol," *Current Opinion in Clinical Nutrition and Metabolic Care* 15, no. 2 (March 2012): 117-21.

Fortuna J. L. "Sweet preference, sugar addiction and the familial history of alcohol dependence: shared neural pathways and genes," *Journal of Psychoactive Drugs* 42, no. 2 (June 2010): 147-51.

Geleijnse, J. M. "Dietary intake of menaquinone is associated with a reduced risk of coronary heart disease: the Rotterdam Study," *Journal of Nutrition* 134, no. 11 (Nov. 2004): 3100-5.

Gilsing, C. et al. "Serum concentrations of vitamin B_{12} and folate in British male omnivores, vegetarians and vegans: results from a cross-sectional analysis of the EPIC-Oxford cohort study," *European Journal of Clinical Nutrition* 64, no. 9 (Sep. 2010): 933-39.

Jacka, F. N., J. A. Pasco, A. Mykletun, et al. "Association between western and traditional diets and depression and anxiety in women," *American Journal of Psychiatry* 167, no. 3 (March 2010): 305-11.

Jacka, F. N., P. J. Kremer, E. R. Leslie, M. Berk, G. C. Patton, et al. "Associations between diet quality and depressed mood in adolescents: results from the Australian Healthy Neighbourhoods Study," *Australian & New Zealand Journal of Psychiatry* 44, no. 5 (May 2010): 435-42.

Jacka, F. N., S. Overland, R. Stewart, G. S. Tell, I. Bjelland, and A. Mykletun. "Association between magnesium intake and depression and anxiety in community-dwelling adults: the Hordaland Health Study," *Australian & New Zealand Journal of Psychiatry* 43 (2009): 45-52.

Jacka, F. et al. "Western diet is associated with a smaller hippocampus: a longitudinal investigation," *BMC Medicine* 13 (2015): 215.

Juanola-Falgarona, M. "Dietary intake of vitamin K is inversely associated with mortality risk," *Journal of Nutrition* 144, no. 5 (May 2014): 743-50.

Hajszan, T. and C. Leranth. "Bisphenol A interferes with synaptic remodeling," *Frontiers in Neuroendocrinology* 31, no. 4 (Oct. 2010): 519-30.

Halyburton, A. K., G. D. Brinkworth, C. J. Wilson, M. Noakes, J. D. Buckley, J. B. Keogh, and P. M. Clifton. "Low- and high-carbohydrate weight-loss diets have similar effects on mood but not cognitive performance," *American Journal of Clinical Nutrition* 86, no. 3 (Sep. 2007): 580–87.

Henderson, V. W., J. R. Guthrie, and L. Dennerstein. "Serum lipids and memory in a population based cohort of middle age women," *Journal of Neurology, Neurosurgery & Psychiatry* 74, no. 11 (Nov. 2003): 1530–35.

Irmisch, G., D. Schlaefke, and J. Richter. "Zinc and Fatty Acids in Depression," *Neurochemical Research* 35, no. 9 (Sep. 2010): 1376–83.

Kennedy, D. O. "Polyphenols and the human brain: plant 'secondary metabolite' ecologic roles and endogenous signaling functions drive benefits," *Advances in Nutrition* 5, no. 5 (Sep. 2014): 515–33.

Lachance, Laura, and Drew Ramsey. "Food, mood, and brain health: implications for the modern clinician," *Missouri Medicine* 112, no. 2 (2015): 111–15.

Lehmann, M., B. Regland, K. Blennow, and C. G. Gottfries. "Vitamin B_{12}-B_6-folate treatment improves blood-brain barrier function in patients with hyperhomocysteinaemia and mild cognitive impairment," *Dementia and Geriatric Cognitive Disorders* 16, no. 3 (2003): 145–50.

Letenneur, L. et al. "Flavonoid Intake and Cognitive Decline over a 10-Year Period," *American Journal of Epidemiology* 165, no. 12 (2007): 1364–71.

Lin, P.Y. and K. P. Su. "A meta-analytic review of double-blind, placebo-controlled trials of antidepressant efficacy of omega-3 fatty acids," *Journal of Clinical Psychiatry* 68, no. 7 (July 2007): 1056–61.

Lukiw, W. J., J. G. Cui, V. L. Marcheselli, M. Bodker, A. Botkjaer, K. Gotlinger, C. N. Serhan, and N. G. Bazan. "A role for docosahexaenoic acid-derived neuroprotectin D1 in neural cell survival and Alzheimer disease," *Journal of Clinical Investigation* 115, no. 10 (Oct. 2005): 2774–83.

Maes, M., N. De Vos, R. Pioli, P. Demedts, A. Wauters, H. Neels, and A. Christophe. "Lower serum vitamin E concentrations in major depression. Another marker of lowered antioxidant defenses in that illness," *Journal of Affective Disorders* 58, no. 3 (June 2000): 241–46.

Miller, A. H., V. Maletic, and C. L. Raison. "Inflammation and its discontents: the role of cytokines in the pathophysiology of major depression," *Biological Psychiatry* 65, no. 9 (May 2009): 732–41.

Michalak, J. et al, "Vegetarian diet and mental disorders: results from a representative community survey," *International Journal of Behavioral Nutrition and Physical Activity* 9 (June 2012): 67.

Morris, M. C., D. A. Evans, C. C. Tangney, J. L. Bienias, R. S. Wilson, N. T. Aggarwal, and P. A. Scherr. "Relation of the tocopherol forms to incident Alzheimer disease and to cognitive change," *American Journal of Clinical Nutrition* 81, no. 2 (Feb. 2005): 508–14.

Morris, M. C. et al. "Brain tocopherols related to Alzheimer's disease neuropathology in humans," *Alzheimer's & Dementia* 11, no. 1 (Jan. 2015): 32–39.

Muldoon, M. F., C. M. Ryan, L. Sheu, J. K. Yao, S. M. Conklin, and S. B. Manuck. "Serum phospholipid docosahexaenonic acid is associated with cognitive functioning during middle adulthood," *Journal of Nutrition* 140, no. 4 (April 2010): 848–53.

Pelsser, L. M. et al. "Effects of a restricted elimination diet on the behaviour of children with attention-deficit hyperactivity disorder (INCA study): a randomised controlled trial," *The Lancet* 377, no. 9764 (Feb. 2011): 494–503.

Ramsey, Drew, Sublette, Elizabeth, and Muskin, Phillip. "Chapter 18: Complimentary and Alternative Treatments." In *Clinical Handbook for the Management of Mood Disorders*. Edited by John J. Mann. Cambridge University Press, 2013, 245–257.

Ramsey, Drew and Phillip Muskin. "Vitamin deficiencies and mental health: how are they linked?" *Current Psychiatry* 12 no. 1 (January 2013): 97–101.

Ranjbar, E., M. S. Kasaei, M. Mohammad-Shirazi, et al. "Effects of zinc supplementation in patients with major depression: a randomized clinical trial," *Iranian Journal of Psychiatry* 8, no. 2. (June 2013): 73–79.

Rivenes, A. C., S. B. Harvey, and A. Mykletun. "The relationship between abdominal fat, obesity, and common mental disorders: results from the HUNT study," *Journal of Psychosomatic Research* 66, no. 4 (April 2009): 269–75.

Rosche, J., C. Uhlmann, R. Weber, and W. Froscher. "The influence of folate serum levels on depressive mood and mental processing in patients with epilepsy treated with enzyme-inducing anti-epileptic drugs," *Acta Neuropyschiatrica* 15 (2003): 63–67.

Rosell, M. S. et al. "Long-chain n–3 polyunsaturated fatty acids in plasma in British meat-eating, vegetarian, and vegan men," *American Journal of Clinical Nutrition* 82, no. 2 (August 2005): 327–34.

Sánchez-Villegas, A., L. Verberne, J. De Irala, M. Ruíz-Canela, E. Toledo, L. Serra-Majem, and M. A. Martínez-González. "Dietary fat intake and the risk of depression: the SUN Project," *PLOS ONE* 6, no. 1 (Jan. 2011): e16268.

Sánchez-Villegas, A., M. Delgado-Rodriguez, A. Alonso et al. "Association of the Mediterranean dietary pattern with the incidence of depression: the Seguimiento Universidad de Navarra/University of Navarra follow-up (SUN) cohort," *Archives of General Psychiatry* 66 (2009): 1090–98.

Sanders, T. A., and S. Reddy. "The influence of a vegetarian diet on the fatty acid composition of human milk and the essential fatty acid status of the infant," *Journal of Pediatrics* 120, no. 4 (April 1992): S71–77.

Sarris, J., A. C. Logan, T. N. Akbaraly, G.P. Amminger et al. "Nutritional medicine as mainstream in psychiatry," *The Lancet Psychiatry* 2, no. 3 (Mar. 2015): 271–74.

Selhub, E. M., A. C. Logan, and A. C. Bested. "Fermented foods, microbiota, and mental health: ancient practice meets nutritional psychiatry," *Journal of Physiological Anthropology* 33 (Jan. 2014): 2.

Sen, C. K., S. Khanna, and S. Roy. "Tocotrienol: the natural vitamin E to defend the nervous system?" *Annals of the New York Academy of Sciences* 1031 (Dec. 2004): 127–42.

Simon G. E. et al. "Association between obesity and psychiatric disorders in the US adult population," *Archives of General Psychiatry* 63 (2006): 824–30.

Slutsky, I. et al. "Enhancement of learning and memory by elevating brain magnesium," *Neuron* 65, no. 2 (Jan. 2010): 165–77.

Smith, A. D. et al. "Homocysteine-lowering by B vitamins slows the rate of accelerated brain atrophy in mild cognitive impairment: a randomized controlled trial," *PLOS ONE* 5, no. 9 (Sep. 2010): e12244.

Solfrizzi, V., C. Capurso, A. D'Introno, A. M. Colacicco, et al. "Dietary fatty acids, age-related cognitive decline, and mild cognitive impairment," *The Journal of Nutrition Health and Aging* 12, no. 6 (Jun.-Jul. 2008): 382–86.

Sommerfield, A. J., I. J. Deary, and B. M. Frier. "Acute hyperglycemia alters mood state and impairs cognitive performance in people with type 2 diabetes," *Diabetes Care* 27, no. 10 (Oct. 2004): 2335–40.

van Gelder, B. M., M. Tijhuis, S. Kalmijn, and D. Kromhout. "Fish consumption, n-3 fatty acids, and subsequent 5-y cognitive decline in elderly men: the Zutphen Elderly Study," *American Journal of Clinical Nutrition* 85, no. 4 (April 2007): 1142–47.

Vogiatzoglou, A., H. Refsum, C. Johnston, S. M. Smith, K. M. Bradley, C. de Jager, M. M. Budge, and A. D. Smith. "Vitamin B$_{12}$ status and rate of brain volume loss in community-dwelling elderly," *Neuroscience Letters* 220, no. 2 (Dec. 1996): 129–32.

Westover, A. N. and L. B. Marangell. "A cross-national relationship between sugar consumption and major depression?" *Depression and Anxiety* 16, no. 3 (2002): 118–20.

Wilkins, C. H., Y. I. Sheline, C. M. Roe, S. J. Birge, and J. C. Morris. "Vitamin D deficiency is associated with low mood and worse cognitive performance in older adults," *American Journal of Geriatric Psychiatry* 14, no. 12 (Dec. 2006): 1032–40.

Wolfe, A. R., E. M. Ogbonna, S. Lim, Y. Li, and J. Zhang. "Dietary linoleic and oleic fatty acids in relation to severe depressed mood: 10 years follow-up of a national cohort," *Progress in Neuro-Psychopharmacology & Biological Psychiatry* 33, no. 6 (Aug. 2009): 972–77.

Wu, A., Z. Ying, and F. Gomez-Pinilla. "Docosahexaenoic acid dietary supplementation enhances the effects of exercise on synaptic plasticity and cognition," *Neuroscience* 155 (Aug. 2008): 751–59.

Yurko-Mauro, K. "Cognitive and cardiovascular benefits of docosahexaenoic acid in aging and cognitive decline," *Current Alzheimer Research* 7, no. 3 (May 2010): 190–96.

INDEX

Page numbers in **boldface** refer to recipes.

D

dairy, 20, 30, 33–35, 60, 74, 95
    calcium in, 73
    complete protein in, 55
    fermented, 95
    grass-fed, 64, 91
    vitamin B$_{12}$ in, 47
dandelion greens, Warm Dandelion Greens with Farmhouse Cheese and Toasted Pine Nuts, **185**
dementia, 9, 16, 17, 20, 33, 37, 42, 50, 57, 58, 61, 72
depression, 9, 14, 16, 17, 19, 20, 21, 37, 41, 42, 43, 44, 47, 49, 50, 52, 57, 64, 66, 87
desserts, recipes for, 259–80
DHA (docosahexaenoic acid), 15, 34, 37, 42, 43, 44, 45, 60, 80–81
diabetes, 4, 5, 17, 43, 48, 62, 64, 71, 103
diseases, 66
    bacteria and, 52–53
    nutrition and, 5, 17, 31
    see also specific diseases
DNA, 21, 40, 44, 45, 46, 49, 50, 54, 66, 67
duck, Pan-Roasted Duck and Potatoes with Cherry Sauce, **232–34**

E

eat complete, 9–10, 17
    brain health and, *see* brain health
    tips for, 22–23
    see also essential 21 nutrients
eggs, 5, 22, 30, 33–35, 43, 55, 60, 89, 91
    Avocado Baked Egg with Roasted Red Pepper Coulis, **124**
    Baked Eggs in Crispy Kale Cups, **126**
    cholesterol in, 96
    Deviled Green Eggs with Roasted Red Pepper and Capers, **153**
    Quinoa-Mushroom Frittata with Fresh Herbs, **120**
    Truffled Farm Egg with Wilted Watercress and Smoked Salmon, **123**
enzymes, 18, 23, 45, 54, 59
EPA (eicosapentaenoic acid), 34, 37, 42, 43, 44, 80–81, 97
ergocalciferol (vitamin D$_2$), 66
essential 21 nutrients, 36–37, 80–83
    for foundation of brain health, 39, 41–56
    for ignition of brain health, 39, 69–79
    for protection of brain health, 39, 57–68

F

fats, cooking, 101, 107–8
fats, dietary, 41–44
    in brain and body health, 12
    fake, 12
    saturated, 21, 41, 64, 95, 107, 108
    trans, 11, 12, 35, 41, 64, 107, 108
    see also omega 3 fats
fennel seeds, 106
    Cinnamon-Fennel Brined Pork Chop with Cauliflower Hash, **225**
fiber, 13, 24, 31, 32, 51, 52, 53, 91, 95, 97–98, 103
fish, 19, 32, 42, 43, 44, 57, 64, 87, 88, 96–97, 101–2
    see also seafood; shellfish; *specific fish*
flavanols, 15, 31
flavonoids, 19, 62
food:
    colors of, 14, 23, 30, 31, 35–36, 62, 63, 89, 91, 94, 108
    diet assessment and, 87–89
    mental health impact of, 3
    organic 30, 36, 63, 94–95, 96, 107
    plant-based, 12, 30–31, 42, 53, 75, 89, 98, 103
    principles for deriving nutrients from, 30–36
    Rules of Kale and, 30
    see also essential 21 nutrients; nutrients, nutrition
free radicals, 18, 39, 57, 78
fritters:
    Double-Green Summer Fritters, **182**
    Millet-Cheddar Fritters over Farm-Fresh Spinach, **138**

G

garlic, 14, 104
    Curried Cauliflower-Garlic Soup with Cashews, **203**
    Garlic Butter Shrimp over Spiralized Zucchini, **246**
    Grilled Wild Salmon with Garlic Scape Pesto and Summer Squash, **245**
    Whole Trout en Papillote with Garlic Broccoli, **249**
gazpacho, Heirloom Tomato Gazpacho, **193**
goat cheese, Black Rice with Grilled Radicchio, Beets, and Goat Cheese, **158**
grains:
    gluten-free 33, 102–3
    refined, 53
    whole, 12, 31, 32, 45, 94
greens, 14, 20, 30, 31, 36, 42, 48, 50, 59, 74, 91, 92, 94
    Bone Broth with Torn Greens, **200**
    Crispy Shrimp with Greens and Beans, **257**
    Double-Green Summer Fritters, **182**
    Kiwi Green Smoothie, **113**
    Lazy Green Mac and Cheese, **162**
    see also specific greens
green tea, 62
    Green Tea Mushroom Soup, **199**

DREW RAMSEY, MD, is one of medicine's leading proponents of using dietary change to help balance moods, sharpen brain function, and improve mental health. He is an assistant clinical professor of psychiatry at Columbia University College of Physicians and Surgeons. In his private practice his work focuses on the clinical treatment of depression and anxiety. Using the latest brain science and nutrition research, modern treatments, and an array of delicious food, he aims to help people live their happiest, healthiest lives.

He is the cocreator of the Brain Food Scale and cofounder of National Kale Day 501(c)3. He frequently speaks and conducts workshops nationally, including two TEDx talks on food and brain health. His work and writing have been featured in the *New York Times*, the *Wall Street Journal*, the *Huffington Post*, *New York Magazine*, *Prevention*, and *Lancet Psychiatry*, and on NPR, which named him a "kale evangelist." His recent bestseller *Fifty Shades of Kale* (Harper Wave, 2013) has made this superfood accessible to thousands. His first book, *The Happiness Diet: A Nutritional Prescription for a Sharp Brain, Balanced Mood, and Lean, Energized Body* (Rodale, 2011), explored the impact of modern diets on brain health.

Dr. Ramsey is a diplomate of the American Board of Psychiatry and Neurology and a Fellow of the American Psychiatric Association. He completed his specialty training in adult psychiatry at Columbia University/New York State Psychiatric Institute, received an MD from Indiana University School of Medicine, and is a Phi Beta Kappa graduate of Earlham College. He lives in New York City with his wife and two children.

Learn more at DrewRamseyMD.com.